"How did globalization shape the COVID-19 pand- COVID-19 pandemic reshaped globalisation? In addressing these questions Chris Peterson presents a comprehensive analysis of the dramatic global social and economic consequences of the COVID-19 pandemic. He surveys in thirteen engaging and accessible chapters how COVID has impacted on the world of work, patterns of inequality, gender relations, technological change, the global political economy and not least climate change. Arguing that the pandemic era is not yet over he offers valuable prescriptions regarding future pandemic management whilst also reflecting upon the significant lessons to be learned from the COVID-19 pandemic for the design of effective global and national responses to the multiple threats and challenges – from the climate emergency to AI – confronting humanity. A terrific contribution to making sense of our era of polycrisis or permacrisis."

Emeritus Professor Tony McGrew, *Strathclyde University, UK*

"Many books on COVID have been written, wondering how, why, and now what. Peterson's welcome and readable retrospect takes a much-needed deep sociological dive."

Emeritus Professor Ronald Labonté, *University of Ottawa, Canada*

Globalisation and Pandemic Management

This book considers the global response on governance after the pandemic while sociologically addressing the effects of COVID-19 on life and work experience.

It presents the effects of COVID-19 on global and local labour markets, the development of digitisation and technology, of work health, and on the environment with respect to global warming and climate change. Linking COVID-19 to the progress of globalisation, the book considers the spread of the pandemic and its management as a response to neoliberalism.

The book analyses national and international governance models for tackling future outcomes of emerging global issues such as technology, green industry and environment that may inform future management of global crises. As such, it will be of interest to scholars in the field of Global Studies, Governance, International Relations, Political Science, Complexity Studies, Environment Studies, Sociology, Disaster Management and Occupational Health.

Chris L. Peterson, PhD, has an Adjunct appointment in the Department of Social Inquiry, La Trobe University, Bundoora, Australia. He specialises in work-related stress, chronic disease and epilepsy and has published extensively in these areas, including several books. He has also recently published the book *Identifying and Managing Risk at Work: Emerging Issues in the Context of Globalisation*. He primarily undertakes quantitative research, but also engages with qualitative research. He is a co-investigator on a six-wave longitudinal study of the social aspects of epilepsy and has been chief investigator or co-investigator on a number of large grants.

Routledge Advances in Sociology

For more information about this series, please visit: https://www.routledge.com/Routledge-Advances-in-Sociology/book-series/SE0511

Globalisation and Pandemic Management

Issues and Outcomes from COVID-19

Chris L. Peterson

Routledge
Taylor & Francis Group

LONDON AND NEW YORK

First published 2024
by Routledge
4 Park Square, Milton Park, Abingdon, Oxon OX14 4RN

and by Routledge
605 Third Avenue, New York, NY 10158

Routledge is an imprint of the Taylor & Francis Group, an informa business

British Library Cataloguing-in-Publication Data
A catalogue record for this book is available from the British Library

ISBN: 978-1-032-58282-5 (hbk)
ISBN: 978-1-032-58284-9 (pbk)
ISBN: 978-1-003-44942-3 (ebk)

DOI: 10.4324/9781003449423

Typeset in Sabon
by KnowledgeWorks Global Ltd.

Contents

Changing impact on globalisation due to COVID-19   97

 9 COVID-19 and climate change   99

10 Growth of the green industry, labour and the
    labour process   110

11 Changes in local, national and global labour markets   122

12 Gender, COVID-19 and changing globalisation   133

13 Labour process and socio-political contexts: A view to
    the future   145

    References   *157*
    Index   *197*

Preface

This book has been written since the declaration of the COVID-19 pandemic in 2020, at a point where it appears to have subsided and most countries have relaxed restrictions. However, the *Lancet*, by 2023, had issued a warning that coronavirus was not over and in China for example early that year there had been mass infections and more than one million deaths in over two months. This was after restrictions had been withdrawn. In late 2023 an eighth wave of COVID-19 was of some concern in Australia. It remains to be seen how this works out. Some had bemoaned dropping mask wearing as a means of mitigating the virus.

As a sociologist I have been engaged in the debate about the relationship between COVID-19 and globalisation. I saw the point in time of the pandemic as an opportunity for the world to reflect on where we had come to with the relatively new phenomenon of globalisation. The 'Spanish flu' around 1918 had more lives lost compared to COVID-19, but coronavirus had substantially many times more economic disruptions and upheavals. My interest has also been in the human side of the pandemic and particularly in some of the very unequal outcomes of the virus and of measures used to contain it. One of the effects of globalisation has been to create some large inequities by race, colour, gender and socio-economic status. The pandemic has reinforced some of these inequities, along colonial lines.

COVID-19 has moved us into the future more quickly, especially with growing technology and digitisation. Home-based work edicts hastened the need to be more technologically literate, with Zoom, Teams and other platforms being required. Also artificial intelligence, surveillance drones and related technologies have been adopted more quickly due to the virus. Some commentators have said the developments have been beneficial while others have reported costs, not the least being increased isolation for certain groups.

Of particular interest to me is the intersection of COVID-19 and global warming/climate change. Together they are of immense concern. With COVID-19 there was a style of governance linking local, national and supranational levels, together with a strong belief in science. These combined with extensive vaccination programmes (although some countries have limited supplies) to respond positively to the threat. Could that same belief in science be harnessed for meeting future possible pandemics and global warming/climate change?

Acknowledgements

This book was born out of an interest, together with many other social scientists, in piecing together a view to the future from a major global crisis. In negotiating the possibility of future pandemics and the reality of global warming/climate change what can be learned from COVID-19 provides valuable lessons. Pathways to successfully dealing with future crises will become clearer with more reflection, investigation and robust debate. What is clear is that under untamed neoliberalism, inequities and vulnerabilities will remain and increase whatever future events unfold depending on the types of governance employed.

I would like to thank my wife Jan Tinetti for providing ceaseless debate and comment over the content of the book. I would also like to thank my long-time colleague Dr Christine Walker and others in the process of producing the book.

The book is dedicated to the frontline health professionals and essential workers who were constantly at risk of infection and possible death due to COVID-19.

Abbreviations

ADR	Autonomous Delivery Robots
AI	Artificial Intelligence
CO$_2$	Carbon dioxide
CSIRO	Commonwealth Scientific and Industrial Research Organisation
DHL	Digital Health Literacy
DRC	Democratic Republic of Congo
EVs	Electric Vehicles
G7 countries	Canada, France, Germany, Italy, Japan, the UK, the US and EU
GFC	Global Financial Crisis (2008)
Global North	North America, Europe, Israel, Japan, South Korea, Australia, New Zealand
Global South	Brazil, India, Indonesia, China, Nigeria, Mexico
GND	Green New Deal
GP	General Practitioner
HSE	Health and Safety Executive
ICT	Information and Communication Technologies
ILO	International Labour Organisation
IMF	International Monetary Fund
IPC	Infection Prevention and Control
OECD	Organisation for Economic Cooperation and Development
OHS	Occupational Health and Safety
OP	Occupational Physician
OSHA	Occupational Safety and Health Administration (US)
PPE	Personal Protective Equipment
PTSD	Post Traumatic Stress Disorder
R&D	Research and Development
UA	Urban Agriculture
UHC	Universal Health Coverage
UN	United Nations
WEF	World Economic Forum
WHO	World Health Organisation

Part I

Introduction

1 Society and its institutions prior to COVID-19

Introduction

In writing this book it is intended to look at globalisation from a point not equalled in its history: the advent of the coronavirus disease-19 (COVID-19) pandemic. The watershed event of coronavirus in late 2019 led to a time of global phenomena emerging, creating a myriad of problems across the world. By early 2023, after three years of COVID-19 there was a sense, in the Western world at least, of some ease, that the peak of the virus had passed. Richter (2022) argues that the period of hindsight creates a challenge as well as the opportunity to research and publish on coronavirus. However, smaller peaks of COVID-19 have occurred, particularly in China, at a time when mask wearing, lockdowns and other measures in many countries including China had ceased. This was a cause for concern. 'The pandemic's residual shadow (apart from its knock-on political and economic impacts) is receding, with the 'slow burn' of antimicrobial resistance and the 'hot burn' of climate change re-emerging as pressing topics in global health governance' (Labonté, Martin and Storeng 2022). There have been threats of new outbreaks and the problem of the 'long-covid' health impact, as well as difficulties in recovery for global health systems. Improvements will need to consider relevant globalisation processes that foster growth and resilience. As late as November 2023 an eighth wave of COVID-19 has had an impact in Australia, albeit milder than previous waves.

By 2024, as the world is recovering from a major catastrophe, this book traces life under the pandemic. It looks at the management of coronavirus by nation states and globally and at how this may prepare us for future global crises. This opening chapter looks at the shape of the world pre- COVID-19, its national and global characteristics, describes the nature of the COVID-19 pandemic, and prepares the reader for the remaining book chapters.

The COVID-19 pandemic plunged the world into a globally threatening crisis, especially between late 2019 and early 2022. A Public Health Emergency of International Concern was issued on January 30, 2000, and a pandemic was declared March 11, 2020 (WHO 2020a). By December 24, 2023, there had been 6,990,067 deaths by COVID-19, 773,119,173 recorded

DOI: 10.4324/9781003449423-2

infections and 13.59 billion vaccine doses given (WHO 2023a). However, there is a concern that official figures grossly underestimate death due to COVID-19. WHO (2023b) reports that from the declaration of the pandemic the death toll rose from 171 to 1,813,188, by the end of December 2020. Yet they claim that deaths due to the virus were 3 million, saying there was a significant undercount of total deaths directly and indirectly resulting from COVID-19. This is because many countries do not have facilities to provide accurate figures. For example, Africa had only 10 per cent capacity to do this.

Society before the pandemic

In the period leading up to the pandemic declaration globally, there had been growth and development, alongside significant drawbacks. Neoliberal globalisation had made countries more than ever dependent on international trade, with supply lines being particularly long. Countries such as Africa were more susceptible to problems of supply. Neoliberalism had been active in increasing inequality and in creating differences in opportunity. There was a significant disadvantage to being of a different race, black, a migrant, and for many women. Vulnerabilities were based on colonial lines (note Bump et al. 2021). There had not been a significant recession in the years before COVID-19, and with free trade agreements, there had been extensive inter-country activity. However, China was starting to restrict trade with countries such as Australia. Environmental issues had become highly visible with problems in gaining agreements to restrict emissions. Weather patterns were changing with mean temperatures increasing. Terrorism and global unrest had increased in part due to the Arab spring and large displaced populations had spread to many areas of the world.

Brexit had occurred in the UK marking their withdrawal from the European Union (MacRae et al. 2021). This affected many UK citizens and significantly reduced some business confidence. Donald Trump the US President was elected with the catchcry 'Make America Great Again.' Tarana Burke had started a social movement, MeToo. Initially it was a rally point for abused and disaffected black women. It later became #metoo, for all affected women (Araujo and Peterson 2021).

COVID-19 impacted on socio-economic, environmental and psychological spheres, and affected many areas of life globally. It has been a testing time for global systems and the processes underpinning them. There was a large risk of economic recession which remains at four years after the start of the pandemic. Pileggi (2021), a researcher from Australia, looked in a systematic way at global performance pre-COVID-19. He combined selected global indices of different aspects of life. Further, he adopted a customised analysis of global development and key priorities which enable a better understanding of times before the pandemic. It also helps to provide a picture of global resilience.

Pileggi (2021) outlines six indicators representing life before COVID-19. The environment and sustainability are represented by global environmental measures (with the challenges of food security and climate change). Health and demographic change (with the challenge of healthcare) is shown by life expectancy. The economy (with challenges of unemployment, global trade, investment strategy, inclusive growth and fiscal crisis) is represented by GPD per capita. In addition, poverty and inequality are represented by the number in extreme poverty. Human rights and freedom (with the challenge of gender equality) are indicated by the number of people living in a democracy. Finally, there is violence and instability, which uses measures represented by terrorism.

The period of global measure referred to is 2000–2015. Positive indicators point to positive global performances and negative indicators, negative performance. Looking at the data reported, health, demographic and life expectancy changes have performed positively; economy (Gross Domestic Product [GDP]) and extreme poverty and inequality, and freedom and human rights have also performed positively. However, environment, sustainability, violence and instability represented by terrorism have performed negatively.

An analysis of data from UN Global Issues identified 22 issues which were negative, but there was reason to be optimistic. The World Economic Forum's (WEF 2019) biggest global challenges were macroeconomic risk, geopolitical and geoeconomic tension, environmental risks, technological vulnerabilities, the human side of risk being mental health concerns, biological risks, and rising sea levels. Borgen Project (2018) is an organisation devoted to reducing poverty. In 2018 it identified ten global issues which had negative performances and there were reasons to have a pessimistic view. These were climate change and pollution, followed by violence and security and well-being; a lack of education, and unemployment was followed by government corruption; malnourishment and hunger were followed by substance abuse and terrorism. Finally, Millennials in the WEF Global Shapers Survey (Kosoff 2017) reported negative performance issues and a pessimistic view. The most concerning for millennials was climate change, followed by large-scale conflict/war; inequality was next, then poverty and religious conflicts; government accountability and transparency, followed by food and water security, a lack of education and safety/security/well-being; and finally lack of economic opportunity and employment.

Overall based on all sources cited, global performance was negative, but the view to the future was optimistic. However, on risks of the future, there was no mention of a pandemic even in the months prior to COVID-19.

The results of Pileggi's (2021) analysis help to bring a better understanding of evolving global developments in pre-pandemic times. He argues that it gives a picture of what may occur post-pandemic. There may be a substantial mindset change bought about by the pandemic that can support sustainable development. It may also lead to a focus on both global institutions and nation states in developing resilience to future pandemics.

Gauging pre-coronavirus times, several pre- and post-virus aspects have affected social and economic structures worldwide. These relate to stress, social influences, threats and moral dynamics in pre-pandemic times. It is expected they will continue post-pandemic (Mishra et al. 2020).

Most countries had large gains in life expectancy in the second half of the 20th century. However, in the beginning of the 21st century, the speed of improvement slowed in several high-income countries, before the coronavirus pandemic. These included England, the US, Scotland and Wales. In addition, the pandemic delivered a substantial decline in life expectancy that many high-income countries had not seen in recent times (Schöley et al. 2022). In 2020 life expectancy in Europe and North America fell by about one year, but in the US it was more than two years. Western Europe in 2021 recovered from losses in life expectancy from 2020. However, Eastern Europe and the US had substantial decreases due to coronavirus for this period. In 2021 most losses overall in life expectancy were due to those registered with COVID-19. In 2022 in Australia female life expectancy reduced by 0.6 years, and males by 0.7 years. The direct effect of the pandemic was about three quarters of this reduction (Adair, 2022).

The role of international organisations in regulating globalisation has been underrated. In the 1980s–2000s there was increasing across border activities involving trade, people and finances. It led to a rapid reduction in global poverty with more than 2 billion people climbing out of extreme poverty by the late 1990s. There were improvements in access to public health, nutrition, employment and sanitation. This led to adding a decade to average life expectancy globally (The Conversation 2020). Worldwide, however, governance by divided nations had been a downside of globalisation. One of its consequences has been the world becoming more interdependent, and that brings certain systemic risks. The Global Financial Crisis (GFC) of 2008 demonstrated this, leading to the prominence of many populist parties. By the time of the pandemic more than 60 per cent of US adults had a chronic disease. One in 8 (or 12.5%) lived below the poverty line and more than 44 million had no health cover. The US is one of only two countries in the Organization for Economic Cooperation and Development (OEDC) not to have Universal Health Coverage (Peterson and Walker 2022). Australia has a strong health system while regions such as Africa, South Asia and Latin America have weak health systems. Faith in a democratic way was at a low point compared to previous decades, remembering that the spread of democracy globally has been relatively recent. In addition, there has been a trust gap between citizens and leaders and a declining trust in leadership. The early presidency of Donald Trump in the US testifies to this (note Peterson 2021a).

Devlin, Fagan and Connaughton (2021) report on a US survey of several countries that were investigated on whether people in advanced societies felt their country to be more divided due to coronavirus: 12 out of 13 developed countries reported less division prior to the pandemic.

The world after coronavirus will not be the same. Reforms are needed to avoid mistakes in future pandemics. Avoiding inequality by listening to all citizens and overcoming divisions can lead to a level of cooperating required to meet the challenges of, for example, future pandemics and climate change (The Conversation 2020). Before the pandemic, economic and social inequality and social problems were high (as well as social pressures) in Organisation for Economic Cooperation and Development (OECD) countries (OECD 2020a) This was despite living conditions improving in the past ten years. Disposable income per capita had increased cumulatively by 6 per cent: however, in Italy and Spain for example it was below 2010 levels. People had problems with falling into a poverty trap. At that time 15 per cent of all full-time workers were in low-income jobs.

Dealing with the healthcare crisis

Petrović et al. (2020) argue that possessing a better prepared health system and having trustworthy organisations affected the outcome of the pandemic. Their study focussed on impact factors in relation to the coronavirus outbreak in 23 European countries. They used a conceptual model to understand preparedness of the existing system. Structure refers to the elements that existed prior to the pandemic that were crucial in ability to cope (including the health system's preparedness for a crisis, and society's coping ability). Process refers to reaction to COVID-19 to reduce transmission and mortality. The researchers (2020) found it was expected that societies with greater capacity to deal with acute crises in health and having greater trust in government and institutions would be better prepared for the pandemic. Yet Petrović et al. (2020) identified that Great Britain, Switzerland, Sweden and the Netherlands, while having advantages over poorer countries, had initial severe outcomes from coronavirus. Slovakia and Italy were the only European countries whose capacity to deal with acute health crises matched the severity of the outbreak. Countries less prepared for COVID-19 (in terms of healthcare systems) and with less trust in government and society's institutions initially performed better. Countries with lower trust appeared to have more prompt and stringent measures against the virus: Eastern European countries had a sharper reaction due to having weaker healthcare systems compared to Western Europe.

Just prior to the pandemic, as late as November 2019 the OECD released their economic outlook. Economies were weak after growth falling to 2.9 per cent during 2019. There was a need to restore confidence and growth including raising living standards. This was due to a slowdown in China and climate change (OECD 2019a). Also, in 2019 a special feature of the Social Outlook (OECD 2019b) was on the LGBT (lesbian, gay, bisexual and transgender) community. Out of 14 OECD countries that kept records 17 million identified as LGTB. Of these one in three reported harassment or discrimination, and they were 7 per cent less likely to be employed.

Park et al. (2021) provided novel data on lifestyle changes in the South Korean population before and after the start of COVID-19. Deterioration in social activities and leisure, nutrition and education led to a more sedentary lifestyle. This led to reduced mental health especially increased depression.

What is COVID-19?

COVID-19 originated in December 2019 in Wuhan city in the province of Hubei in China, On January 30, 2020, WHO said the coronavirus was a worldwide crisis severely affecting humans (Mishra et al. 2020). Early in March 2020, the WHO declared COVID-19 a global pandemic. In the preceding fortnight outside of China there was a 13-fold increase of cases, and there was a three-fold increase in the number of countries reporting infections (Cucinotta and Vanelli 2020). In China those infected had a diagnosis with symptoms including headache, fatigue, intense respiratory disorder, headache, fatigue, mild fever and throat pain (Mishra et al. 2020).

COVID-19 is an infectious disease due to the SARS-Cov-2 virus (WHO 2023c). People infected mostly experience mild-to-moderate respiratory symptoms and recover without the need for special treatment. Others get seriously ill and need medical intervention. Those more likely to develop a serious illness were older and having conditions such as diabetes, cancer, chronic respiratory disease and cardiovascular disease. Anyone can get unwell, or seriously ill, or die. COVID-19 has affected health and has been a reason for an increased death rate around the world. There have also been financial and political crises in countries affected as well as major economic and social costs (Mishra et al. 2020).

WHO (2023a) report in August 2023 the top ten countries for number of infections were the US, followed by China; India, France and then Germany; and Brazil, Republic of Korea, Japan, Italy and the UK. The highest number of deaths is in the US, Brazil and India, followed by Russia and Mexico.

To deal with containing the spread of the virus, there are several precautions based on what was mandated by government. These included physical distancing from others being 1.5 metres to stop the spread of droplets; deep cleaning surfaces in public areas; the wearing of masks in public, including in taxis, on other public transport, and in the height of the pandemic at home; lockdowns were amongst the most severe measures, to a small radius from home; curfews; and no travel unless essential. These restrictions were difficult for many people (note Margaritis et al. 2020). The co-workers maintain that young people may appear protected from the virus, however prolonged lockdown creates risks to their health and well-being. Being sedentary for extended periods can lead to cardiovascular and other problems for all people. As a means of long-term control and containment, vaccines were administered in many countries late in 2020.

Despite coronavirus being more than three years old, a warning has been issued. The Lancet (2023) argue that the crisis of COVID-19 is not over:

far from it. The global response is inadequate and fragmented, despite three years of experience and 'international treaties of pandemic preparedness. In 2023, far from it being the end of the pandemic (as hoped by many and announced for the USA by President Biden in September ... 2022), there is a new, dangerous phase that requires urgent attention' (The Lancet 2023, 79).

In late 2022 China dropped most of its restrictions with the virus, possibly as a reaction to their stringent zero-COVID policy. Quarantining was relaxed and lockdowns were generally not needed for municipal areas or cities and were less stringent. International travel resumed. By the end of 2022 millions of Chinese had been infected. There were narrower definitions of infection and deaths used for reporting. Chinese people entered a difficult phase by 2023. The vaccination rate, particularly for older people, has not been adequate: a vaccination drive was initiated. The Lancet (2023) outlined that celebrations of the Lunar Chinese New Year may have spread infections to rural regions. Internationally, strong travel restrictions have been in place, but these may have counterproductive consequences. 'Rather than hoping for the end, letting our guard down, and thinking that the problem is somewhere else, everyone needs to remain alert; encourage maximum transparency in reporting cases, hospital admissions, and deaths; and accelerate collaborative surveillance of variant testing and vaccinations. The pandemic is far from over' (The Lancet 2023, 79). Du et al. (2023) estimate that after the December 2022 relaxation of restrictions in China, there were 1.41 million deaths between December 2022 and February 2023. This was much higher than reported officially.

WHO declared an end to the COVID-19 disease on May 5, 2023. Lee et al. (2023), however, report there are new coronavirus risk variants and case numbers and deaths remain. SARS-CoV-2 remains a serious threat, particularly with potentially new variants emerging.

Further chapters in the book

Summaries of the remaining 12 chapters follow.

Introduction

Chapter 2 presents an overview of globalisation and the impact of COVID-19. The relatively short period of modern globalisation is discussed, as is the contribution of a sociological perspective. A brief history of globalisation is presented: Bryan Turner maintains globalisation is an all-embracing paradigm in sociology. He says it is feared more than being understood. Ulrich Beck has defined globalisation and risk as one of several features of modernity. He presented a rather pessimistic view of the welfare state, and this has been challenged by several writers. COVID-19 has seen many nations expanding the welfare state (albeit temporarily) to avoid fiscal devastation. Further sociological approaches to the study of globalisation are detailed. The later part of the chapter focusses on the impact of the pandemic and how this has affected globalisation. Vaccination issues are also discussed. The virus has had a major impact on tourism, supply chains, international commerce and higher education. Finally national contributions to researching coronavirus are outlined. It has been argued that COVID-19 could lead to a new growth or an adapted mode of globalisation.

Chapter 3 presents the bases of neoliberalism. That is, how it developed and what conditions sustain it. It was first expressed in the 1930s and developed through the 1940s–1960s. The relationship between neoliberalism and globalisation, and a political economy approach is presented. There have been a number of sociological studies of neoliberalism and much has been made of inequity under neoliberal governance. Ulrich Beck has described a growing inequity; however, critics have argued this is more a case of the rich getting much richer. Beck also discusses individualisation, where people are shouldering the burden of precarious work, unemployment and underemployment. Vincente Navarro has criticised several international organisations for promoting neoliberalism. COVID-19 and its relationship to neoliberalism are also outlined. Navarro maintains any government using neoliberal policies and practices to combat the coronavirus is extremely foolhardy. Studies in sociology, including political sociology, help explain the relationship between science and neoliberalism There are links drawn between industry and academic research with the regulation of technology by science discussed.

Specific effects of COVID-19

The relationship between the COVID-19 pandemic and globalisation is discussed further. Chapter 4 investigates whether what we have learned will bring about a better world. Inequality is one of the greatest outcomes of COVID-19. Globalisation itself has had effects on COVID-19, and some writers maintain that globalisation, through the proliferation of urbanisation, international trade and opening of national borders, has been a breeding ground for the transmission of pathogens. COVID-19 has also had substantial effects on globalisation. There has been the shortening of supply chains, and difficulty in protecting workers in many industries, particularly front-line health and mobile workers. Some have argued that COVID-19 has had effects on globalisation, from 'bending but not breaking,' to entering a period of 'deglobalisation.' Meeting the challenges of climate change may require similar styles of governance to dealing with COVID-19. There has also been a greater trust and reliance on science. A question is how could climate change be approached with a similar trust in science? Effects of COVID-19 on the labour process are discussed. For some, albeit higher socio-economic employees, much work became home-based leading to additional scrutiny of the home by management, sometimes leading to alienation of workers from their everyday lives.

There are several approaches to understanding occupational health and safety (OHS) including a focus on socio-political perspectives. In Chapter 5 it is argued that an emphasis on OHS over the past three decades has been on growing numbers of organisations utilising precarious work. The growth in precarity during globalisation has been extensive, replacing post World War 2 stability in employment. Labour markets are now characterised by underemployment and less secure work. In terms of OHS risk, Europe has reported that stress is the second highest occupational illness and injury. With COVID-19 there has been an unprecedented burden on healthcare and on economies. Morbidity and mortality of workers due to COVID-19 largely followed pre-pandemic patterns of inequity. Many mobile workers have experienced high risks of infection due to poor cramped working and living conditions. In addition, frontline health workers were up to three times more likely to be infected, and in many cases there had been an under supply of protective equipment. During coronavirus OHS had an important role in providing advice on safe ways of working. COVID-19, lockdowns and the possibility of recession have led to increased health inequalities.

Chapter 6 starts by discussing the state of economies during COVID-19. Coronavirus has had an extensive impact on national finances and economic performance. It has also had a major influence on how we live and work. Technology is having unprecedented effects. For many, work became home based using online technologies. Even after the peak of the virus, much work has become home based with hybrid option being used. This has placed a premium on learning to 'Zoom' or use 'Teams' to substitute face-to-face interaction. It has meant many workers have had to upgrade skills with information and communications technology (ICT), and much monitoring has created problems. Working from home can reduce the support base and create social and mental health problems which require maintaining healthy routines. COVID-19 has changed the use of technology, much of it in healthcare. People needing more sociability and interpersonal contact have reported stress. During 2020 the flexible working patterns that could have produced greater well-being and productivity happened much more quickly than expected.

We have moved into an age where technology has become dominant, the age of digitalisation. In Chapter 7, according to Ulrich Beck the dominant forces of science and technology are important components in risk society. Richard Baldwin discusses digitalisation, automation and 'globotics.' Baldwin argues that many workers involved with ICT have increased their control over their jobs due to upgraded technical skills and expertise. Labour process involving technology and the increased use of metrics is further discussed. There are three sociological perspectives discussed for understanding digital technology: political economy, Foucault and 'more than human' approaches. The use of metrics is a way of recording outputs and productivity of workers, and its increased use can lead to a decrease in power and control of workers. As a result of COVID-19 sharing information is a requirement, and information transparency and acting collectively have been essential in dealing with the pandemic. The use of technology and digitisation have increased enormously because of COVID-19 with changed work patterns for many.

The focus of Chapter 8 is on the global effect of coronavirus and its management, and outcomes for the world. The OECD is cited in there being heterogeneous effects of the crisis with financial, health and economic consequences. A move towards authoritarianism, inequality and misinformation after the virus has been predicted. National and subnational government organisations have dealt with 'territorial effects' of coronavirus. The main social and economic implications of coronavirus are presented. Deprived areas have been more affected and in the US late in 2020 rural counties had higher death rates. There was massive fiscal support for households, businesses and the vulnerable, and large investment recovery initiatives by some governments. One outcome was the use of financial incentives by governments to support their citizens who had lost their jobs. In some countries there was a brief return to the welfare state. Additionally, there was considerable inter-government cooperation at various levels in the state and with international bodies. The caution is that the neoliberal model is not suited to or effective in dealing with the pandemic. Coronavirus had contributed to social inequality which may become more evident after recovery, although debate on this is polarised. There were several mandates by government some of which have longer-term implications.

Changing impact of globalisation due to COVID-19

Public health is concerned about how climate change and the pandemic intersect. Chapter 9 starts by looking at the UN global approach to climate change. There has been concern about global warming/climate change for some decades. At a global level, despite planning to reduce emissions there has not been significant agreement until recently when most countries moved to support major planned reductions. The consequences of global warming are extreme weather events with the likelihood that poorer countries would endure the worst outcomes. Further, the effects of the pandemic on global warming/climate change are outlined. For a time during the pandemic, there was a significant reduction in emissions. Theoretical approaches to climate change based around Ulrich Beck's *Risk Society* thesis are discussed. Ways, including through imagination, are posed to find solutions to the global crisis. There are several issues of governance employed with COVID-19 which can contribute to managing climate change. While much of the management of climate change needs to be carried out at local levels, if governments are not involved sufficiently then measures may not succeed. There also needs to be governance at the national, inter-government and supra-government levels.

Chapter 10 starts with the edict that to become resource efficient and have a low carbon economy, countries need to change. Agriculture, energy and waste management use a lot of resources and have high emissions. Resource efficiency needs to increase. In the US 19.4 per cent of employed workers could be working in the green economy (this would include indirect green jobs, not needing high knowledge or skill changes). A labour process analysis looks at some transitions to green industry. Electric vehicles are an important commodity for the future but with green technology there are some anomalies. Cobalt mining in the Democratic Republic of the Congo is carried out in sometimes slave like conditions to provide for advanced batteries amongst other things. Green jobs also may provide greater control opportunities for workers, but that depends on the level of automation. COVID-19 has bought about a rethink of the globalised social and economic models derived from neoliberal globalisation as countries moved through the coronavirus. Green financing, green bonds and technology impact on UN CO_2 targets. Lessons learned from global cooperation in COVID-19 and issues of governance become planning benchmarks for expanding a green economy.

Risks involved in modernity and the nature of work including precarity have been discussed by Beck. In Chapter 11 these arguments are critically appraised. Labour markets have been undergoing transitions during recent times. Before COVID-19 there was globalisation, technological change and automation, and the creation of green industries. This signalled a divide where cities benefitted from these changes, but other regions did not. In the US 13 per cent of people are working in jobs which didn't exist in 1970. The labour market is likely to become more skilled because of COVID-19, but one sector that diminished during the pandemic is universities. COVID-19 reduced their growth due to the lack of international education and in countries such as Australia government did not financially support university jobs. The education of many younger people due to the virus has been delayed by uncertainty and lack of opportunity. The other disadvantaged group are the unskilled precarious workers which have grown during the pandemic. By four years after the start of the pandemic some countries were experiencing labour shortages.

Prior to COVID-19 there were changes to gender relations that saw inroads towards what appeared to be some equity in the workplace. Chapter 12 identifies that in the previous decade social movements had given women in some countries a voice that had long been suppressed. The most public of the social movements was 'Me Too' (with Tarana Burke) (also #metoo) in the US which became a forum for all women to express acts of gender harassment. Beck's risk society is discussed and critically evaluated in relation to gendered inequity. The effect of COVID-19 was to emphasise existing gendered inequities, with women being worse off overall than men. It halted progress to gender equality and increased the division of labour, unemployment and reduced working hours. Job loss worldwide for women was 1.8 times that for men. Women accounted for 39 per cent of employment; however, they represent 54 per cent of job losses. More women engaged in unpaid care. In North Africa, South Asia and the Middle East, women perform 80–90 per cent of unpaid work. Acting on gendered inequity could lead to improving the lives of millions of women and stimulate global economic growth. The upsurge of violence against women during lockdowns is also discussed.

Chapter 13 presents a labour process approach in discussing a changing social, occupational and economic landscape, because of COVID-19. Ulrich Beck's *Risk Society* thesis is discussed and evaluated in the context of socio-political consequences of the virus. A labour process approach looks at the edict of working from home. One aspect of moving through the pandemic and new forms of globalisation is that an understanding of socio-political factors and of political economy is essential. The effect of coronavirus on political economy has been great. It mirrors patterns of resource extraction whose foundations are colonialism, marginalisation and racial discrimination. There are lessons learned about national and international governance. The book finishes with a consideration of how we can apply what we have learned from the COVID-19 experience to other global threats such as future pandemics and global warming/climate change. The pandemic has drawn a global response in protecting nations as economic responses included increasing welfare to deal with the economic fallout. The forms of governance used may be suitable for future global crises. A belief in science has fuelled the response to COVID-19: could this same belief translate into addressing climate change?

Conclusion

Prior to the COVID-19 pandemic the world had experienced economic advances and improvements in health and medical systems, and in health indicators such as life expectancy. While globally there had been improvements these had been overshadowed by increasing inequities, between those with resources and power and those without. Many of these differences were on colonial lines. Neoliberal globalisation, based on the rule of the market, had exacerbated these differences. There have been warnings issued that COVID-19 is still present and that vigilance is needed. Respiratory effects may be lasting.

Issues such as impending global warming/climate change were needed to be dealt with and these require a political will and global unity. COVID-19 was not anticipated and delivered a major shock to nations and globally. The hope is to learn from the governance of the pandemic.

2 Globalisation and sociological contributions
The impact of COVID-19

This chapter begins by exploring the historical roots of globalisation. While regarded as emerging in the 1980s, globalisation and its practices were evident in the mid-19th century. Ulrich Beck outlined globalisation and risk as an outcome of modernity with both positive and negative effects. Sociological approaches to studying and understanding a global world are discussed. Following this there is an analysis of the impact of the COVID pandemic on a globalised world and contributions to researching the virus.

Historical bases of globalisation

Alcalde and Escribano (2020) report that several sociologists have traced the beginning of globalisation back to the 16th century or earlier. However, Gulmez (2017) maintains that research on global activity was as early as the 15th century. Beck (2000a) reported a few possible starting dates with modern capitalism, and Giddens (2000) refers to characteristics of globalised society existing in the late 19th century. Northrup (2009) argues that the Industrial Revolution around 1800, maritime expansion by the West about 1500 and Asian integration around 1000 represent the three most likely starting times of globalisation. Economists tend to identify a later starting date and historians an earlier one. Williamson (1996) outlined three stages of globalisation, and these came after the mid-19th century: the late 19th century; between the beginning of World War 1 and 1950; and then in the late 20th century. The period during the 19th century appears to have most currency.

Lecler et al. (2019) argue that the terms 'global' and 'globalisation' have changed from not existing before 1980 in scientific publications to being explosive in several disciplines. These included economics and sociology. Some have argued that Marx analysed the growth of capitalism in the mid-19th century, and this had many aspects of contemporary globalisation. At that time there was expansive capitalism, increases in international trade, production dispersion, foreign investment and the growth of 'economic interdependence.' There are communication, information and cultural aspects, and 'it… promotes the rise of a global and mobile bourgeoisie, while increasing

DOI: 10.4324/9781003449423-3

and reinforcing world inequalities' (Lecler et al. 2019, 358). Globalisation has socio-economic, socio-political, and sociocultural elements all captured by a sociological perspective.

Globalisation and risk

Globalisation has become an all-embracing paradigm in sociology, and sociology has a prominent voice in the field (Turner 2010a). He maintains that globalisation theory has moved from economic systems, through culture into political systems such as global governance (Turner 2010b). Part of the background of globalisation is in the prevailing culture and consciousness that have spread throughout the world. Beyond inequality, Turner (2010a) points to global ethics. A possible future for globalisation is a 'feral society of urban decay' with wars about water and pandemics, or it could be a bond around 'shared cosmopolitan ethics.' Turner (2010b) says globalisation is feared more than it is understood.

Haberland (2009) uses a Marxist framework in referring to global dominance that is implicit in globalisation. Beck (2000a) refers to establishing cooperation and 'dependencies at a distance' under globalisation. Globalism was an ideology for rule by the world market – that of neoliberalism. Globalisation is evident in attempts to minimise damage from coronavirus disease-19 (COVID-19). Nation states have been active in mitigating the virus' effects and developing global cooperation replacing intensely competitive relationships between nations.

Thorpe and Inglis (2019) argue that young people now have the technology to share social, cultural and political challenges. Social media, such as Facebook, helps young people to form alliances in difficult situations. They can directly share their experiences. Mass movements such as #metoo (Araujo and Peterson 2021) and Black Lives Matter have also been a binding force for young as well as old based largely around social media. Bryan Turner, Ulrich Beck and Elisabeth Beck-Gernsheim, in the context of social movements, argue that young people are a group forming a single 'global generation' (note Beck and Beck-Gernsheim 2009; Edmunds and Turner 2002).

Contributions of Beck

Beck's work highlighted contemporary issues and amplified fears about globalisation and risk. It focussed amongst other things on global ecology, pandemics and the consequences of exposure to technology. Beck commented about mediation on markets, and science and technology under modernity that are shaping the spread of capitalism. He said that global outcomes 'are undermining their own benefits' or have the potential to do so (Jarvis 2008).

'Modernity itself, according to Beck …. has created a world of uncontrollable risks (e.g., financial, ecological, and terrorism) and potential catastrophes, which neither respect state boundaries nor are clearly tied to one actor or source' (Zhou 2022, 453). Ulrich Beck recognised that risk is increasing due to developments in science, industrialism and technology. Later modernity created greater risk, not less. He felt globalisation challenged the 'sovereignty of the nation-state' and leads to the reduction of the state's authority while compromising 'economic sovereignty.' This happens because of following 'the whims of mobile capital' (note Jarvis 2008). Markets become denationalised and global. The state's response is international. Citizenship in this process is less democratic, and accountability and probity are compromised. The partial erosion of the state is seen to be due to globalisation.

There is a 'power play' between governments, unions, parliament and citizens which is not territory based. These include trade, finance and capital resulting in 'political economic uncertainty and risk' (Beck 1999). In the past three decades the welfare state has been 'rolled back' due partly to reduced corporate tax levels. The unemployed, disabled and destitute are not properly supported due to its demise. The state passes its responsibilities on to individuals who become responsible through self-protection, increasing the risks citizens take (for example, with disability insurance and the use of savings).

Beck discussed 'individualisation' which represents the way that many workers need to take responsibility for their employment and the risk that is involved. They also need to reinvent themselves to meet the changing demands of the workplace and of capital. An example is 'gig' workers who are employed precariously and must work as independent contractors with no sick or holiday leave entitlements. It also applies to many migrant workers during COVID-19 who had no access to healthcare or government benefits, even when working in 'essential' jobs. The diminishing welfare state has left many people unemployed or underemployed.

According to Beck the progress of science entails greater risk. The response to COVID-19 has seen a widespread belief and trust of science (except for conspiracy theories and misinformation on social media platforms). Coincidently this deeper trust in science has not translated into trust in the science of other crises such as global warming/climate change.

Beck was concerned with globalisation and its effect on the state's capacity to function effectively. That is for institutions to have enough capacity to perform and for the state to be autonomous. He claims sovereignty is surrendered by cultural change, economic processes and political means. A focus on 'risk society' is important for sociologists looking at COVID-19. It concentrates on social change and structure (Ward 2020). How does the non-discriminating virus (where risk is seen as democratic) affect some groups more than others because of different material circumstances? Disadvantaged and more at-risk groups can include those engaged in precarious employment and living in slums or other circumstances. This challenges some pretexts of risk society.

Jarvis (2008) argues that Beck's depiction of globalisation is rather negative (although others do not share that view, note Guivent 2016). With Beck's proposition of states offloading responsibilities onto individuals, in many cases state taxed income has increased for countries during globalisation. However, there are several globalised corporations such as Apple, Microsoft and Facebook that pay little or no tax. Beck asserts that in a hollowing out of the welfare state there are indications that state fiscal capacity has increased during globalisation. In addition, the advent of the COVID-19 pandemic shows that under dire threat a number of nations are prepared to expand the welfare state to avoid fiscal devastation.

There is greater discretionary spending by states, and any decline in welfare spending is more likely not due just to globalisation. States have more flexibility than proposed by Beck. He overstated globalisation, especially about capital mobility and that capital 'deserts the state' leading to fiscal crises (Jarvis 2008). In addition, rather than creating increased risk for capital, it remains constant in developed countries. There is not much evidence showing structural change in the global market value locus of the largest corporations. This is less than Beck's theories might indicate.

Globalisation has occurred by the state's local actions and what causes globalisation is opposite to that maintained by Beck and general 'globalisation theorists' (Jarvis 2008). This suggests under globalisation states have done quite well with capital accumulation. It had significant growth (between 1970 and 2004) that contrary to Beck's proposition, we are now seeing the nation state as growing in security and economic protection. That is, it is growing stronger under globalisation.

There is little evidence supporting Beck's idea that states are retreating, with the erosion of their fiscal bases. In Organisation for Economic Cooperation and Development (OECD) countries, fiscal bases have increased as globalisation continues. Jarvis (2008) also questions Beck over claims that globalisation has diminished political strength and welfare. This is contrary to what Beck proposed as globalisation impoverishes lower groups in society, and incomes of the rich have increased. The individualisation of risk through reduced welfare or tax systems under globalisation might not be automatic.

In later work Beck (2011) argued that transnational companies outsource jobs to countries with cheaper labour and that international competition from all kinds of workers has reduced. Outsourcing capitalism produces competition between foreign and domestic labour. He says that this creates 'a coercive cosmopolitisation unfolding.' This can be seen in the proliferation of mobile workers in regions such as South Asia, Southeast Asia and Canada during COVID-19 (see Neis et al. 2021 on the susceptibility of mobile workers in Canada to infection and death). The vulnerability of outsourced and mobile workers is up to the domestic state governments to guard and treat, as globalisation retreats due to coronavirus.

According to Beck many problems such as climate change need global solutions. States are not equipped to solve such problems. They need global governance called 'cosmopolitan democracy.' Martell (2008) argues these global issues will need a consideration of differing power relations and conflicting interests and these happen at the level of nation states. Global cooperation is also essential. In many countries action initiated on climate change is occurring at a greater degree of governance closer to the ground.

Jarvis (2008) discussed economic outcomes of globalisation. This was through such things as relocating capital from 'core to periphery,' from Western European factories to the sweatshops of developing countries. Beck had little opportunity to look at global financial organisation and its product of increased precarity. At this point in history precarity is a major aspect of the organisation of labour, argued to provide employers greater flexibility to increase profits for shareholders.

Nonetheless there has been a steady growth of globalised corporations which form the basis of the globalised economic community. Some future problems, such as pandemics and global warming/climate change, need global governance to ensure that countries' territorial and local issues do not dominate decision and policymaking.

Other sociological approaches to globalisation

Theories of globalisation have been debated extensively but with the onset late in 2019 of coronavirus some of the basic tenets of neoliberal globalisation have been undermined. For example, it has been considered entirely inappropriate in dealing with the pandemic. Some claim that globalisation will not return to its lofty levels pre-COVID-19. Others claim globalisation may disappear. Whatever happens it is unlikely to be the same as pre-pandemic.

Romain Lecler et al. (2019) discussed the basis of a renewed interest in studying globalisation. They claim globalisation had begun mid-19th century and argue that sociological globalisation theories of the 1990s moved the focus from a national to global level. There were six aspects of contemporary globalisation presented by sociologists. These are the invention of 'globalisation' and 'global' terms; the development of 'transmigrations'; emerging international trade, 'value chains,' and logistics; 'global cities' and new 'transnational financial flows;' the threat of globalised culture to 'cultural diversity;' and a more widespread and ordinary sociology of globalisation.

'The very notion of 'waves' of globalisation supported the sceptics' thesis that globalisation is just a myth .... For example, they argue that transnational corporations ... are neither new nor particularly numerous. They assert that globalised capital remains concentrated in developed countries, as well as the bulk of trade, investment, and financial flows, as it was before' (Lecler et al. 2019, 356). Globalisation as a term now encompasses phenomena going way beyond increasing international trade and refers to qualitative and quantitative changes in how international exchanges are carried out, affecting societies globally.

Many sociologists have focussed on the novelty of globalisation with the most influential theories being developed during the 1990s. According to Lecler et al. (2019) new issues emerged, including communication and transnational media, epidemics and studies of the environment. Sociologists have looked at 'global ethnography' (note Gille and Riain 2022), transnational phenomena such as migration round trips, border issues (note Fauser, Friedrichs and Harders 2019), 'global policies' (Engel and Burch 2021; Maire 2023) and the forces of capitalism (Robinson 2018). Globalisation has encompassed issues way beyond opening international trade. It refers to changes in international exchanges, their conduct and how they affect societies around the globe.

Lecler et al. (2019) published on globalisation and what makes globalisation new two months before the COVID-19 outbreak was reported in China. The point being that an analysis of sociological perspectives took place on globalisation at the point where a global catastrophe would re-write some of its rules, heading into a new world order. There may be a return to previous levels of globalisation post-pandemic, but not in the immediate future. Some have called COVID-19 the beginning of 'de-globalisation.' Some ask the question '(I)f globalization is a new phenomenon, what does it comprehend, and why are the social sciences better equipped to analyse it?' (Lecler et al. 2019, 355).

Labonté, Martin and Storeng (2022) maintain that globalisation is not dead or dying. It has been in different forms for 5,000 years, the most recent iteration being neoliberalism since the 1980s. They raise several questions on whether globalisation as we know it has been dealt a death blow. Factors are COVID-19, the Russian war in the Ukraine, the war between Israel and Gaza and 'a breakdown in multilateralism.' Does this mean returning to the 'stagflation of the 1970s?'

The first year of the pandemic saw persistent reductions in global trade's value with restrictions on goods needed for the COVID response. Global supply chains are vulnerable to any shocks such as coronavirus. Rich countries during the pandemic did not agree to 'any meaningful waiver of the WTO TRIPS rules' (involving limitations on exports) which could help poorer countries access vaccines and other health commodities. This could affect trade reforms in the future.

COVID-19 is bringing about changes to globalisation that will be long term. Ciravegna and Michailova (2022) observe three trends. These are, inequalities have increased, both within and between countries; nationalism and populism have also increased; further, anti-globalisation feelings have intensified due to strains undermining institutions which have promoted globalisation. These factors have bought about growing uncertainty. This includes a reconfiguration of value chains resulting from increased costs and has led to a partial retreat from globalisation to a more regionalised economy. COVID-19 has severely affected globalisation by disrupting international trade (Mena, Karatzas and Hansen 2022).

'The unravelling of the COVID-19 pandemic in 2020 has forcefully remarked the relevance of social reproduction as a key analytical lens through which we can interrogate and analyse contemporary capitalist processes, their features, outcomes and crises' (Mezzadri, Newman and Stevano 2022, 1783). The co-workers show how reproductive dynamics represent the 'everyday' in a global economy in several ways. These include the state and provisions of care, work in labour processes, paid and unpaid work, and global processes of everyday social relations.

Pieterse (2008) writing more than a decade and a half ago forecast the rise of China, East Asia and India as another rejigging of capitalism and 'relocation of accumulation regions.' He maintained that the inclusion of these areas is related to neoliberalism. Martin, Metzger and Pierre (2006) report that two of the distinct subjects of the sociology of globalisation are, firstly, defining 'global' and secondly identifying changes in most countries. They draw on social movements and a 'sociology of the elite' to help explain power and power differentials. There is a need for accurate and reliable data. 'We try to identify, then explain, social processes common to (almost) all countries of the world (or more accurately, common to all relevant entities) and which are 'going in the same direction' (Martin et al. 2006, 503). They argue that the study of globalisation refers to global social phenomena and results from processes gained from a range of global organisations, global movements and transnational corporations. Sowers (2017) discussed what she refers to as a neglected aspect of globalisation – the rise of the logistics industry. The researcher argues that logistics workers are in a very powerful position in that the 'logistics revolution' plays a key role in the capitalist system. The workers have a 'structural brokerage' role in the worldwide economy. Political movements may well capitalise on their position. The workers need to be understood as potentially powerful in the context of globalisation.

Raab et al. (2008) developed an index for measuring globalisation. There has been an emphasis on grand theories in defining globalisation in sociology. When researchers assess the presence of globalisation or if it is a new phenomenon, and how it impacts on life in industrialised societies, we need to be more precise in specifying globalisation. Economists have provided more specific definitions. Raab et al. (2008) identified four dimensions of globalisation: economic, socio-technological, cultural and political. They say the index is based on a genuinely sociological analysis.

Pauwells (2019) proposed a visual identity approach to recording cultural elements of globalisation, as part of a series of indicators of degrees of globalisation. This focusses on material culture as well as human public behaviour in urban contexts to enrich 'more abstract discourses on globalisation.' This is based on using grounded data. For example, Coca Cola, Apple, Facebook, Microsoft, McDonalds and other related identifying cultural elements can be used as urban visualisations of material culture relevant to globalisation. Global problems such as COVID-19 and climate change need global cooperation implying transnational solidarity. Pauwell's approach provides a refreshing addition to studying globalisation with qualitative and mixed methods tools which go beyond the many economic analyses of the phenomenon. It represents a constructivist and metaphoric approach.

Another qualitative study, utilising narrative interview methods, was conducted on the social aspects of face mask use during COVID-19 (Hanna et al. 2022). Many other studies of masks have focussed only on the technical aspects in relation to protecting from disease transmission. One aspect of their study was the potential stigma and exclusion experienced due to intolerance of those who did not wear masks. Small-scale sociological studies influence policymakers on the impact of COVID-19 on sociopsychological and economic effects, particularly on families and households and transmission of the virus within households (Hantrais et al. 2022). These same studies can contextualise human experience and reaction in the context of an altering globalisation during the pandemic.

Sociology and COVID-19: Trends and vaccines

COVID-19 is a social event beyond being medical that social scientists and sociologists are well equipped to study (Deflem 2022). Methodologically, however, opportunities to conduct face-to-face fieldwork were severely limited by the virus, while online connections with individuals and families grew and flourished (note Hantrais et al. 2022).

Jeanne et al. (2022) maintain that the danger of the SARS-COV-2 has been enormous. Spanish Flu took about a year to become global whereas COVID-19 took two months to affect the 'main centres of globalisation.' The virus led to rivalry between nations unable to deal with the impacts on health. There were tensions between developed countries related to accessing health and medical resources. This needed to signal a warning in relation to the progress of the virus in developing countries such as Africa, Latin America, South and Central Asia and the Middle East. It has become clear that the spread of coronavirus is at different speeds in different countries. Developed countries and China have focussed on dealing with the virus spread while others have been unable to provide required assistance to regions such as Africa.

According to Zhou (2022) around August 2020 the richest countries had reserved sufficient COVID doses of vaccine to immunise their populations many times over while poorer counties had limited access. He reviewed literature on vaccine nationalism. Firstly, there were global tension such as between the US and China before the pandemic. Considering also the Global Financial Crisis (GFC), these factors help to explain why COVID vaccines and the WHO became the sites of global competition. Zhou maintains vaccine nationalism involves 'geopolitics, international economic inequalities, global capitalism, and 'me-first' politics' (2022, 451) In addition there is the COVID-19 Vaccines Global Access (COVAX) which responds to vaccine nationalism, showing the nature of a globalist approach creating equal access to global goods. Vaccine nationalism has shown the dangers of nationalist responses to global emergencies and shows where action is needed with contemporary globalisation. This suggests that with non-economic issues global cooperation is not achieved effectively.

Katz et al. (2021) writing more than one year into the virus say that for many poorer countries, vaccine distribution does not exist. Eighty per cent of these populations may not receive a vaccination into the second year of the pandemic. This has made ending the virus more difficult. Apart from distribution there are other barriers to uptake, including misinformation, mistrust and confidence in vaccines. Even wealthy countries have barriers to effective campaigns, but vaccine nationalism leads to a great price paid by poorer countries.

A study of 48 European countries showed those with stronger globalisation have gained from higher rates of vaccination (Lupu and Tiganasu 2022). Those countries more economically open and with more integration with international marketplaces might be able to access vaccine suppliers more quickly. The co-workers argue that globalisation's effect on vaccination is indisputable. Internationally opinions, knowledge and best practice need to be shared. More developed countries allocate more funding and resources to respond to crises, gaining faster access to vaccines and vaccination programmes. Countries in the European Union (EU) are in a favourable position, and the governance develops the confidence of citizens in accepting vaccination. Countries with greater globalisation are more diversified and can withstand greater and more varied 'shocks.'

Puri et al. (2020) describe the role that social media has played in promulgating anti-vaccination messages. These have promoted a degree of hesitancy about vaccination, and they argue it leads to a compromised public health confidence in preventing COVID-19. There is an 'irreversible trend' in the roles of digital technologies and social media in vaccination. There are issues of ethics to be addressed and the digital divide which influences health inequities (Zang et al. 2023).

Sociology: Other aspects of coronavirus

Lusardi and Tomelleri (2020) proposed that COVID-19 is a 'breaking point' of culture. They considered it 'a watershed' of a social order spanning the last 40 years, and the order to come. It has become evident that this pandemic has no equal in our recent past. That is the global extent of its spread, the restrictions on personal freedoms, the extent of the economic crisis and the duration of the emergency. The authors (2020) sought to raise questions on the economic, sociocultural and technological aspects of the virus to imagine future occurrences. The sociological bases are those that drove modernity. According to Beck (1992) the potential of 'instrumental rationality,' the driver, was also a base of modernity. It had many risks: unlimited trust in experts and in technical/scientific progress, as well as the desire to control nature and social processes.

Although it appears there had been insufficient planning for adverse events, in fact there have been extensive amounts of economic and social planning (Lusardi and Tomelleri 2020). The co-workers maintain the forces behind modernity have improved billions of lives and made an evolutionary leap for our species, taking the 'planet into the Anthropocene era.' Interdependence between family, education, economy and politics does not mean risk is eliminated. Despite increases in prediction by scientific and technical models, events may not be entirely predictable as humans are a dependent and variable part of those systems. The neoliberal economy has a fast-evolving technology. The emergence of COVID-19 was an unseen and unexpected side effect of our model of development (note Beck 1992). It has challenged neoliberal globalisation. Over an indefinite period, there have been consumption and productivity downturns, social isolation and making futures difficult to predict. We are like our ancestors. Due to the freedom and wealth of the second half of the last century we forgot our roots and it appeared these 'enemies' of humankind had 'been defeated forever' (Lusardi and Tomelleri 2020).

The COVID-19 pandemic was a profound crisis (Matthewman and Huppatz 2020). With lockdowns and enforced isolation it involves an experiment, one that needs a sociological analysis. Meeting the challenges involves unparalleled surveillance and gendered effects. However, on a positive side, there has been welfare reform, although in some cases temporarily, and universal basic income appears a possibility in some regions.

Ward (2020) argues that there are two avenues of debate for sociologists in relation to COVID-19. One is government policy focussing on health and/or wealth. This refers to questions of political economy including dealing with physical distancing and closing businesses, and increased unemployment. In addition, there is policy on controlling the virus spread, and in trust in the government for the future. There are also issues of tension between government and their citizens in looking after health and wealth. There is the issue of social bonds being weakened by physical distancing. Does it lead to fear of the 'other?' Ward (2020) claims do we 'other' all of those apart from those we live with? Will post-COVID-19 be more individualistic? Research is also needed on how the media portrays COVID-19. Does it mean there will be a greater trust in science than before the virus?

Nygren and Olofsson (2020) critically analysed the 'soft' approach taken by the Swedish government to managing COVID-19 in the initial stages of the pandemic. Their analysis was based on Beck's risk society thesis. According to Beck (1992) risk society rests on several mega risks that threaten humanity, globalisation, dependence on experts and scientific knowledge, individualisation with the replacement of social class and risk positions with inequity remaining. The situation in Sweden where managing the pandemic was based on individual responsibility and expert judgement reflects Beck's risk society of a globalised economy. However, are there still class and gender inequities or are these 'individualised risk positions?' Based on Foucault (1976) 2003 it may be possible to see

Swedish pandemic management as 'governing of contact and individual responsibilisation,' an approach historically based in the welfare state of Sweden (Nygren and Olofsson 2020).

Mansouri and Sefidgarbaei (2021) describe how Beck's (2000b) concept of 'reflexive modernisation' helps to identify where unpredictable and unintended effects of modernity take place. COVID-19 is a disease of risk society, represented by 'border fading' in all countries. It has distance aspects, time and social dimensions. The disease is not localised, has no boundaries and is truly globalised. COVID-19 has a long incubation period and control processes, including vaccination, having long-term consequences for the world. Socially it is one of the most momentous events this century in causing major social stress and disrupting social interactions.

Walby (2021) identified neoliberal and social democratic perspectives of forms of governance. These are behind early debates about authoritarian and libertarian ways of managing the pandemic. Public health is a social democratic approach by states. Walby argues that public health represents an important moment between neoliberal and social democratic approaches and governance. Public health is a social model where efficiency and justice are linked. Neoliberal interventions can create minimalist outcomes. Public health should not adopt authoritarian methods.

Contributions to the study of COVID-19

Worldwide scientists raced to gain an understanding of SARS-CoV-2, so they can develop interventions to control the virus. 'Scientists typically work quietly at a planned pace, but the COVID-19 pandemic altered the priority, methodology and speed by which science is conducted, communicated and translated' (Kana, LaPorte and Jaye 2021, 1). Indications are that the spread of the virus in Africa has been slower and less severe than other regions, but more epidemiological data is needed. Based on a review of the literature, Africa had contributed three per cent of all publications on COVID-19 ten months into the pandemic. Kana et al. (2021) argue that in the long term African scientists require collaboration in boosting scientific productivity.

Worldwide the US represented most collaborations, followed by the UK. In further detail a review of 7,185 publications on COVID-19 (about one-third articles) was undertaken by Grammes et al. (2020). The most involved three countries were the US, China and then Italy. There was a correlation between COVID-19 cases or deaths with research output for the region. The US shared mainly with the UK, as well as China and Italy. China collaborated most frequently with the US, then the UK.

In another report on COVID-19 research activity the EU, US and China produced the largest number of COVID-19 research articles. This was based on a study of more than 18,000 scientific papers (Naujokaityte 2020). Each region published about one-third of the articles. Members of EU states made the largest contribution on how COVID-19 interfaces with diabetes and cardiovascular disease, crisis management, neurology, economics and model-ling, as well as vaccines, therapeutics, and the health effects of the virus.

Zyoud (2021) reported on the research productivity on COVID-19 from December 2019 to March 2021 by the Arab world: 4.26 per cent of the global output of research documents were undertaken (n = 6131). Approxi-mately 65 per cent were journal articles and 16 per cent reviews. Saudi Ara-bia published the most (35.65%), then Egypt (20.78%) and United Arab Emirates (UAE) (11.73%). Controlling for population and GDP the most output was from Saudi Arabia and UAE followed by Lebanon. Later, Al-Bloushi (2022) reported that Saudi Arabia ranked 15th in the world for COVID-19 publications.

Kuipers, van der Witt and Wolbers (2022) undertook a bibliometric re-view identifying themes related to COVID-19 in disaster and crisis literature. They found issues such as governance, vulnerability, resilience, risk and risk communication were raised. New issues such as state power, citizen behav-iour and mental health and business also emerged. There have also been several studies looking at lessons learned through COVID and how to deal with pandemics in the future.

Conclusion

There is a need to articulate a sociological perspective when addressing globalisation, given the history of sociological research on the topic. It is uniquely placed in the context of the pandemic. Globalisation was identified by Marx in the mid-19th century: it has developed extensively in the past few decades to become an all-encompassing issue affecting most layers of society. Understanding the role of risk in modernity is a valuable tool of analysis and Beck's work points to a future, with the growth of science and technology, at greater risk.

Until the onset of the COVID pandemic, globalisation had achieved very high levels of interdependence, of trade and development albeit at a cost of extreme inequities. Some commentators now say we may not return to the heights of transnationalism experienced before COVID-19. A key question is 'can we return to the principles and practices pre the pandemic,' or as some argue have the ground rules changed and are we operating through a new set of local, national and global standards?

3 Neoliberalism in a new order

This chapter outlines the origins of the neoliberalism concept, how it developed and the conditions under which it is sustained. The barriers that exist and the factors that enable the growth of neoliberalism are presented as well as the relationship between neoliberalism and globalisation. Further, there are relevant sociological studies discussed, as well as those about inequity resulting from neoliberalism. Much has been made of the outcome of inequity. The factors behind inequity and its principal indicators and their measurement are examined. The effect of coronavirus disease-19 (COVID-19) on neoliberalism as well as the role of science in sustaining it is presented.

The neoliberal concept

When discussing the political economy of development in scientific discourse the neoliberalism concept is problematic. It has many contradictory meanings. It has also created a divide between the rest of the social sciences and economics. Venugopal (2015) argues that neoliberalism is neither everywhere nor nowhere. It is the dominant economic approach in our time – a powerful political agenda about class exploitation, being 'an overarching dystopian zeitgeist of late-capitalist excess' (2015, 165). Since the 1980s the use of the term has expanded exponentially. Is it a 'paradigmatic' departure, or a 'recalibration' of the relationship between state and market relations? For Venugopal a key question remains: can an all-embracing concept serve in all situations? Neoliberalism is 'a crisis ridden term' due to conceptual ambiguity.

Early neoliberalism derived from the Paris organised 'Lippmann Colloquium' in 1938. According to Brennetot (2015) at that time it was a 'geopolitical doctrine' redressing the world's 'spatial fragmentation into states.' Neoliberalism arose as a political system with territories submitted to a free 'multilateral' division of labour. Neoliberal ideology gained importance later because of a 'neoliberal thought collective' (Sims et al. 2022), based on the work of Friedrich Hayek, and tied to Milton Friedman. This has been very influential.

DOI: 10.4324/9781003449423-4

In the field of moral economy, Hayek saw positive effects on values of particular social institutions (Rodrigues 2013). He was sceptical of market societies' future as seen in institutions having detrimental ideas about markets. He saw deliberately shaping public opinion as important. In 1947 he established the Mont Pelerin Society, including Karl Popper, Frank Knight, Ludwig von Mises, George Stigler and Milton Friedman. They formed a defence of classical liberalism including individual freedom (Peters 2022). It was against totalitarianism and in opposition to Marxist and Keynesian growth of the state.

Ibled (2023) argues that cruelty constitutes neoliberalism from its inception. The author argues that the brutality of neoliberalism is a natural evolutionary outcome of the development of civilisation according to Friedrich Hayek. Two of his early writings were Hayek (1945), where he looked at problems of a rational economic order, and Hayek (1948). His approach has been claimed to have eugenicist undertones. The cruel methods referred to are said to be eliminating bad practices and habits. Hayek has gendered assumptions that lead to 'hegemonic masculinities' in neoliberalism (Garlick 2023). Neoliberalism emerged in the 1930s and 1940s as a set of views preparing for a 'new political doctrine' which allowed the social order to be fashioned by 'individual actions' based under a price system (Colin-Jaeger 2021).

Neoliberalism gained popular use as a term from 'left-wing commentators' late in the 1970s as a pejorative description for free market approaches used by Margaret Thatcher and Ronald Reagan, respectively from 1979 and 1980 (Peters 2021a). It represented policies focussed on 'deregulating capital markets,' globalised 'free trade,' and privatisation based on assets selling off from the state. Conservative and right-wing governments reduced state powers including welfare provisions. Neoliberalism was a shift to a free market orientation. 'Financialisaton is a... term that has its origins in Marxist theory but became an increasingly popular term in the critical literature after the Global Financial Crisis (GFC) after 2008 to refer to the development of financial capitalism in the period after 1980 when increasingly financial markets and financial institutions, encouraged by neoliberalism, became dominant in education and social life' (Peters 2021a).

According to Nicolescu and Neaga (2014) neoliberal policies appear related to both democratic, authoritarian, and even totalitarian rule, while they are most often associated with 'transnational corporate' entities, financial organisations internationally and 'the globalisation process.' Neoliberalism is a concept operating in a de-regulated political sphere (Becchio and Leghissa 2016). They claim it is not a natural extension of old classical liberalism. Neoliberalism represents the dominance of a free market economy, as is usually associated with Western societies.

From the 1940s and 1950s with the proliferation of welfare states some argued that totalitarianism would come out of state intervention. Milton Friedman was one in the 1960s who disagreed that intervention by government could improve 'economic performance.' He spoke out for markets and competition and reducing the state's role (Barnett and Bagshaw 2020). This led to increasing efficiency and productivity and became known as neoliberalism. Milton Friedman also wrote on freedom requiring capitalism (Friedman and Friedman 2002).

COVID-19 shows how inequality is reproduced by neoliberal economies. Neoliberalism refers to free market policies, involving little government spending or control, and low taxation levels. Generally, it is seen as leading to increasing economic and social inequity (Peterson and Walker 2022; Walker and Peterson 2021). The pandemic has led to nine million dying (WHO 2023a). This may be an underestimate. Those of colour, race and lower socio-economic status have been most affected.

Neoliberalism and globalisation

Ulrich Beck describes the world as globalised through neoliberalism. Capital is mobile and the neoliberal world is both instable and interdependent (Martell 2008). To deal with problems of magnitude we need to go beyond the nation state. He suggests a move from neoliberal globalisation to global governance. Winder (2011) writes that in Beck's *Risk Society* (1992) neoliberalism did not appear. Beck, in discussion, did not see 'neoliberal marketisation' resolving challenges posed by risk society. He saw that global risks were breaking down challenges to states' abilities to manage environments, markets and societies. In Chapter 2 of this volume Beck's position on globalisation is discussed as it relates to neoliberal tendencies of reducing the welfare state and to the upsurge in precarity in labour. He has described a growing inequity; however, critics have argued this is more a case of the rich getting much richer. Beck also discusses individualisation, where people are shouldering the burden of precarious work, unemployment and underemployment.

Navarro (1998) critically evaluated the development of neoliberal policies. He looked at the neoliberal belief that the economy in the US is highly efficient and the EU economies are debilitated due to being welfare states with rigid labour markets. He argued that some countries have lower unemployment levels than the US and cites the weakening of the labour movement and power of financial markets as two causes of polarisation between nations. Neoliberal policies on deregulating the labour market led to labour force instability and to worsening living conditions for most.

Neoliberal policies overseen by the International Monetary Fund have led to corrupt practices in political capitalism in developing countries, according to Reinsberg, Kentikelenis and Stubbs (2021). They discuss Max Weber (2001) in that 'politically determined capitalism' with 'politically privileged monopoly industries,' involves colonialism and the 'extraction of hyper profits.' Ayres (2004) refers to the rise of the anti-globalisation movement and identifies several neoliberal short comings.

Neoliberalism and inequity

Neoliberalism threatens democracy by reducing social regulation and hampering policy. In another context democracy may be a threat to neoliberalism. Neoliberalism affects those protecting small producers, policies protecting stability and providing employment, and jobs of the lowest paid workers. The reduction of control by the state in the west from 1980 has led to a substantial increase in wealth inequity (Olssen 2004). In studies of neoliberalism in India there is a tendency to focus on it as a 'hegemonic ideological project' (Baru and Mohan. 2018). Some of these studies have examined the roles of the International Monetary Fund (IMF) and World Bank in extending neoliberalism in India.

Writing in 2013 Koechlin argues that the US story is not just about unemployment, declining incomes and stagnation. It is also about the rich having a robust economy after the GFC. In 2010 in the US the richest one per cent had 93 per cent of the income growth. Since the early 1980s income and wealth inequity in the US have grown, with the state becoming less aggressive in addressing it. It has also become less effective and less generous (Koechlin 2013). He claims the US is the' most unequal' amongst rich countries. Economic mobility has the US nearly bottom of the list, and this is in times of social and political inequality.

In a Marxist analysis Tyler (2015) argues that the meaning of the term class is inequity. The names recorded in the history and geography of class, such as the rich, elites and working class refer to 'structural conditions of inequality.' This is the basis of neoliberalism around the globe.

Watson (2016) argues that several 'cross-national studies' from the late 1990s demonstrated that in most western countries inequity had grown, especially amongst those fully espousing neoliberalism. After being complacent about the connections between inequality and 'free' markets even the OECD started warning that economic inequality was bad in creating economic risk leading to political 'instability.' In several instances inequality had replaced a trend towards increased equality that occurred since the Second World War. Growing inequality appeared to mirror the degree of neoliberalism. In the US and UK, the extent of inequality was large and sudden. However, Watson (2016) argues that in countries such as Canada and Sweden the growth was more modest.

From the 1960s, those supporting neoliberalism have used wealth to develop organisations that foster the free market ideology. This is where the poor are penalised and wealthy rewarded (Dewey 2017). Now neoliberalism appears to be the normal condition. Under Ronald Reagan (1981–1989) as President of the US the difference between the top 1 per cent and bottom 10 per cent of Americans expanded from 65 times as great to 115 times. Regan had enforced large tax cuts and reduced government programmes as well as wages for poorer workers, while investor profits increased. After Regan left office the gap in wealth increased substantially.

Barnett and Bagshaw (2020) argue that neoliberalism as a form of socio-economic and political institution needs challenging: many accept it as the natural order. Gross discrepancies in wealth versus poverty exist around the globe. Many of the differences follow traditional colonial routes, with several nations being unable to catch up to the wealthier regions of the world. Some claim that while inequity has increased, those in poverty have improved their lot, albeit marginally. Yet the costs of inequity will continue to be borne by the less well-off through exploitation. There are also national health costs associated with unequal relations in work and healthcare.

Neoliberalism is based on the belief that progress and well-being are the increased responsibility of individuals, 'entrepreneurial freedom' and increased free trade: this is while keeping government involvement at a minimum. Neoliberalism can be harmful because it promotes competition, leads to undermining social security and a sense of solidarity (Becker, Hartwich and Haslan 2021). Under neoliberalism, economic differences are seen as due to 'differences in hard work.' Inequity represents a deserving difference. The study of social psychology on neoliberalism is new. However, social scientists have shown that inequality can negatively affect imprisonment rates, educational achievement, violence and obesity as well as mental and physical health (Becker et al. 2021). Yet impacts on loneliness and isolation due to neoliberalism have been under-studied.

There are questions in education about neoliberalism's effects on policy and practice. Patrick (2013) argues that by not exploring these effects neoliberal ideology will become entrenched, and education will have mainly functional outcomes. She discusses how globalised neoliberalism interfaces with the knowledge economy and how neoliberal policy shapes learners. There needs to be further consideration of the place of neoliberalism in educations' aims and policies. It sees students' roles as becoming future workers and treats education as a 'means to this end.' Toquero, Calargo and Pormento (2021) argue that neoliberalism has corroded the ideal of 'equality and popular sovereignty' in distance education. It has placed economic and political restrictions on the medical workforce as well as in education. Jarvis (2021) has argued specifically about the effects of neoliberalism on universities and of how the continued use of managerialism and metrics as well as other surveillance methods have seriously eroded academic freedom and the educational experience. Croucher and Locke (2020) suggest that coming out of COVID-19 there needs to be an evaluation of the future of higher education in Australia, so that mistakes of the past are not repeated. There has also been a shift from 'nationalist language ideologies' in TESOL (teaching English to speakers of other languages) literature. This has produced a neoliberal area of study that fits an economic and political context of our period. It relates to flexible workers performing technological jobs as part of 'a post Fordist political economy' (Flores 2013).

Sowles (2019) argues that inequality in the Anglophone world played an important part in the emergence of 'populist political movements.'

This created nationalist and protectionist politics, particularly in the UK and the US. In both countries, globalisation and neoliberalism have enhanced negative feelings against 'metropolitan elites' and the 'status quo.' He argues that Brexit and the rise of Donald Trump in the US were outcomes of these negative sentiments particularly since the GFC (note Peterson 2021a).

Neoliberalism and COVID-19

Briggs, Lloyd and Telford (2020) argue that neoliberalism, despite much criticism, has been 'stubbornly resistant' to change. It promotes the market as the solution to recalcitrant problems and endorses consumer spending as economically necessary, having satisfying subjective outcomes. Just after the transatlantic banking crisis (GFC) neoliberalism was described as 'dead but dominant.' There had been riots opposed to neoliberal capitalism, but neoliberalism asserted its dominance. One commentator suggested that a global catastrophe is the only thing that would lead to change. One such event arrived late 2019 with COVID-19. Briggs et al. (2020) assess the meaning of this for democracies in the western world as they attempted to reconstruct their economies following the 'catastrophic event.'

Globalisation is the outcome of the move towards neoliberal policies based on market reforms since 1970 (Quiggin 1999). One major effect of the pandemic has been the shortening of supply chains. Free and Hecimovic (2021) investigated the effect of COVID-19 on supply and demand, with the disruption of global supply chains. They argue that accounting techniques and 'rhetoric' have ingrained the vulnerability of supply chains during COVID-19. Post-pandemic, the authors (2021) argue accounting procedures may develop more robust supply chains.

Untamed capitalism would represent a foolhardy approach to dealing with COVID-19 (Navarro 2020). Sumonja (2021) argues the pandemic does not mean the neoliberal age is over due to global governments falling back on Keynesian approaches. There was a market versus state dichotomy occurring. There have been emergency conditions, where the state undertakes to do whatever is necessary to stop the breakdown of the current social order. The state has organised the 'neoliberal assault' on all obstacles to the profits of 'capital accumulation' (Sumonja 2021).

Navarro (2020) argues that a key element of neoliberalism has been how 'large pharmaceutical companies' behave in primarily prioritising their maximisation of profits over, for example curing illness which may spread into pandemics. The commercialisation of medicine and putting private before public interests have affected quality of life and health negatively for millions of people. Major policies of neoliberalism include mass privatisation of medical care. Trump, argues Navarro, was the major proponent of this approach. 'Neoliberalism became the hegemonic ideology of both national and international institutions such as the World Health Organization, International Monetary Fund, World Bank, Central European Bank, European Parliament, and European Commission (among many others) ... that facilitated the expansion of the current pandemic' (Navarro 2020, 271).

The advent of the pandemic challenged the long period of austerity and public service cuts in the UK as well as the period of small government in the neoliberal state (Cooper and Szreter 2023). Globally states had intervened comprehensively with coronavirus stirring up notions of the 'role of government.' In the UK the 'hands off' government prepared inadequately to meet the virus. Cuts to the public sector compromised the effectiveness of health services. Those most vulnerable had an increased exposure to risk of dying.

In Brazil during COVID-19 social movements were targeted, there was a reduction of social participation in managing the state, and inequality deepened using extensive neoliberal measures. According to Moura de Oliveira and Verissimo Veronese (2023) the relationship between the authoritarian style of President Bolsonaro and the placing of market interests at the cost of thousands of lives and misery created for many was due to an ultra-neoliberalism style of government. They claim he failed to inform the public and provided misinformation, spreading 'false and contradictory' material. This spurned chaos as well as conflicts between the population and local administrators such as governors and mayors, and with health providers. A damaging path of neoliberalism was the result.

Sumonja (2021) argues that during coronavirus neoliberalism was disintegrating 'in real time': reflected in state against market as a 'shift in power.' Saad-Filho (2020) refers to the virus as the greatest economic collapse under capitalism. The demise of neoliberalism can be looked at as a shift in power with the state in favour (Monbiot 2020). According to Giroux (2021) COVID-19 has been both an ideological and political crisis. Neoliberalism represents a destructive assault on the community. Neoliberalism ruled when in March 2020 US President Trump called to 'reopen the economy,' from Easter. Neoliberalism also brought about an attack on the welfare state.

Some countries in North America and Europe performed poorly with COVID-19 infections and deaths, despite regarded as the most capable of withstanding the pandemic. The US and the UK were ranked as best prepared by The World Economic Forum's Global Security Index (Jones and Hameiri 2021). Yet they were the worst performers. In addition, Britain has Universal Health Coverage (and the US is one of only two OECD countries who do not) (Peterson and Walker 2022). Therefore, why did the UK perform so badly? Other countries which ranked as best prepared but experienced very high death rates were Italy, Spain, France and Germany. Jones and Hameiri (2021) argue that in the move towards neoliberalism, 'governance' has replaced 'government' where authority has been gained by various public and private entities. State managers only assumed a 'regulatory' role. They coordinated negatively to point these entities in 'favoured directions.' An outgrowth has been 'meta-governance' at global and regional levels, with international institutions aiming to blend 'domestic regulation' based on 'shared international principles' and 'best practice.' This includes entities such as WHO's International Health Regulations. The state failed in the context of COVID-19 to address serious societal challenges.

Neoliberalism has led to deteriorating health services during coronavirus (Chalk 2021). It has focussed more on profitability than health indicators, limiting access to health services and health quality that people can afford. Crouch (2022) argues that COVID-19 has allowed time to reflect on the importance of public services and that employees require security and opportunities for collective action. This could form the basis of the will to address greater challenges such as climate change. However, there will be conflicts over whether neoliberalism allows these changes.

At this point in time after the coronavirus peak, primary healthcare is extremely important, but is 'in need of revitalisation' (Mhazo and Maponga 2023), especially in low- and middle-income countries. This particularly is the case in Southeast Asian and African countries. Recently due to the pandemic efforts to increase primary healthcare have been related to increasing Universal Health Coverage and Global Health Security, which emphasise care for those who cannot afford it. This is so households can access medical care when they need it. It is important to support primary healthcare that has endured four decades of neoliberal globalisation, emphasising individual responsibility for health and a reduced reliance on the state. Mhazo and Maponga (2023) argue that primary healthcare has lost its momentum over the years, culminating in a crisis during COVID-19. Social justice paradigms have dominated but need to be reformulated under health security.

Ageing effects

In the UK 89.3 per cent of deaths from coronavirus in the first wave were older people (Shimoni 2023). In March people aged 70 years and older were told to self-isolate for an unknown length of time. However, it was not clear what government policy would address managing this risk. In March 2020 providers of aged care services were told to reduce caring for their needs. Aged care was to be used to house older patients to 'free up National Health Service (NHS) capacity.' Shimoni (2023) reported policy-based negligence in treating older people. Under neoliberalism there has been individualising of health and other aspects of life which make older people more vulnerable with less support. The researcher undertook a newspaper analysis on the depiction of older people in the UK. The risk of infection and dying was seen as unmanageable. Depicted as such undid protection of these people from COVID-19. Older people were 'unseen' and 'unprotectable.'

Barriers to health

Peters (2021b) argues that prior to coronavirus many of those in 'neoliberal debt economies' were living 'hand-to-mouth' with few savings. The virus made the 'debt crisis' immediate. COVID-19 has had a major effect on 'human capital,' learning, well-being and productivity.

'Neoliberal capitalism' is a barrier to effective COVID-19 action (Mair 2021). Private capital is not sufficiently responsive in dealing with changes. By producing exchange through monetary value 'neoliberal capitalism' has developed a barrier to producing 'health value,' and consequently left many countries poorly prepared for COVID-19. Mair introduced concepts of an 'ecological, feminist, and Marxist perspective.' The economy produces goods and services; neoliberal capitalism creates a priority for exchange value which has led to unprecedented productivity; this capacity produces increased exchange value and undermines other values such as health. Successful responses to COVID-19 prioritise life and health and 'undermine exchange value.' For the future, nations need to construct economies that can recognise many 'forms of value.'

Tooze (2021) maintains that in earlier pandemics, the scale of global response was nothing like in 2020. All countries (rich and poor) paid a high price. By April 2020, much of the world was fighting to combat the virus. Lockdown was the term used most. Armed police patrolled the streets in cities in India, France and South Africa. One per cent of the Dominican Republic population were arrested for breaching lockdown. Consumers stayed at home, businesses shifted to being home based or closed, and shutting down became the norm. Those outside their countries such as many thousands of seafarers as well as large numbers of mobile workers became stranded in a limbo (note Neis et al. 2021).

COVID-19 hit worldwide at a time when economic imbalances, political upheavals and financial crises were evident. Global neoliberalism relied more on violent duress since the GFC, resulting in crises in democracy and an increase in authoritarian styles of government (Saad-Filho 2021). At times, leaders had the support of mass movements, with some being far-right groups (in Brazil, India and Donald Trump in the US for example) (note Peterson 2021b). There were measures to create economic stability under extreme neoliberalism such as 'fiscal austerity' which involved punishing the poor and disadvantaged.

Exposure to hazards

Dutta (2020) argues that the housing of low wage migrant workers in Singapore during COVID-19 exposed them to health hazards. This was a case of authoritarian neoliberalism. Singapore's used authoritarian techniques to control labour, and this is based on generating profits under 'extreme neoliberalism.' It was the 'Singapore model.' It used coercive policies based on surveillance and everyday violence. In extreme neoliberalism, violence and authoritarianism interact and are normalised through 'everyday acts of communicative inversions' (deviation into the unexpected) (Dutta 2020).

The pandemic's emergence and the rise of increasing globalisation, social insecurity and economic inequality have led to the failures of 'planned resilience' for profit medicine and making health market based. This is rule by the market. Thereby COVID-19's damage has intensified (Sparke and Williams 2022). Other forces at work were 'structural racism' and 'colonialism,' which are basic to the political economy. COVID-19 provided evidence that neoliberalism has bought about 'health-damaging changes' in the international order of globalisation. The researchers (2022) argue that neoliberal practices and policies in pursuit of wealth have had a negative effect on health during the virus. They call 'socioviral co-pathogenesis' a 'neoliberal disease.' COVID-19, they and many researchers maintain, has been found to fall short in a market-driven world 'body politic.'

The pandemic has exposed the toxic effects of a system that has for far too long dominated every aspect of our societies. Neoliberalism had reduced public services, made education and healthcare profit-based, promoted profit at the cost of underpaid and undervalued workers. It has promoted being militarised compared to human well-being and inequality (Isakovic 2021). Coronavirus demonstrates the main effects of neoliberalism. Gender, race, class and age underwrite how being isolated due to the virus can be carried out: whether work can be done at home, how healthcare can be accessed and whether finances are adequate. Employment has reduced; the care burden of women has increased; and mobilities affected. The researcher (2021) continues that even though the scale will be different after coronavirus, the problems will be similar in future. We can use the momentum of change to transform the operation of societies.

Resilience is required, as the crisis is compared to endurance and its effect on the 'reproduction of neoliberalism' (Damar 2023). There need to be new political options in relation to the pandemic. Neoliberalism is seen to represent injustice and inequity. The researcher (2023) maintains that coronavirus has not heralded the death or indeed the regeneration of neoliberalism. In looking at labour in Turkey under COVID-19 he identifies how the state, organisations and certain workers 'regenerate' the bases of neoliberalism. That is by deregulation, increased competitiveness, individualism, flexibility of the labour market and in seeking status.

Hall (2022) argues that many researchers have discussed coronavirus without considering the context of the broader economy. However, COVID-19 and the GFC, neoliberal austerity and climate change are important considerations. The 'deglobalising' effect of the war between Russia and Ukraine has meant that our thinking should include the changing nature of neoliberalism and the socio-economic and political context of coronavirus. The war between Israel and Gaza adds to the complexity. These factors would then provide a lens through which vital global factors could be appraised for their role in the development, or reconstitution, of neoliberalism.

Neoliberalism and science

Moore et al. (2011) link several approaches in sociology (including political sociology and the theories of social movements), to explain the relationship between science and neoliberalisation. These present a background to transformations between science and scientists. This allows links between industrial and academic research; the increased regulation of technology in trade by science; and the growth of the relationship between publics and scientists. It forms the groundwork for the role of science in neoliberalism.

The three components in Brazilian education to emerge in curricula are meritocracy, competitiveness and individualism. The neoliberal ideas in education counteract against inequality (Vilanova, Miranda and Martins 2021). Nicolescu and Neaga (2014, 104) investigated 'neoliberal policy outputs in Romanian higher education, and also the way in which neoliberalism has become an embedded ideological structure' in higher education. Neoliberalism in universities emerged during the 1970s and 1980s as their market orientation changed with budgetary cutbacks. As the market-based approach developed, scientific research depended more on commercialisation. In Australia more than three decades ago the CSIRO (research organisation) altered funding to support scientific research that had commercial applications, a move away from previous pure science research. This thereby represented the commodification of science and scientific research.

COVID-19 as well as climate change have led to questioning scientific knowledge. Davi et al. (2021) argue the key reasons are due to the application of neoliberal concepts to research. With neoliberalism research has shifted from independent research teams with established jobs, to project teams with 'non-permanent scientists.' It has changed scientific knowledge to being based on 'managerial evaluation of science,' built on 'bibliometrics and quantitative indicators,' and based on 'publications and citations.' This is rather than 'the quality of scientific questions' or the 'continuity of scientific careers.' Jarvis (2021) also argues this in noting the changing management of university jobs and careers and their evaluation. Davi et al. (2021) argue further that the COVID-19 and climate change crises should provide opportunities to emphasise the role of scientists and to ensure they operate in public organisations, where they do not need to bow to conflictual private interests.

Conclusion

In summary, neoliberalism as a concept emerged prior to the Second World War, developed between 1940s and 1960s, but gained traction in the late 1970s and early 1980s. It's base as being market driven has had an enormous global impact, but its consequences in terms of inequality have been far reaching and have created a host of problems. Since the time of Ronald Regan in the US and Margaret Thatcher in the UK the market has been the base for economic and social planning. However, COVID-19 represents a global crisis that neoliberalism could not deal with. Government intervention was needed as a protection enabling a pathway through the pandemic and providing important lessons for future global crises, such as other pandemics and global warming/climate change.

Neoliberalism, in the face of major global threats, will not disappear, but it may change and adapt for more effective future social planning, particularly in tackling growing inequality. During COVID-19 many countries returned to welfare policies to combat health and economic crises. This may be a path to adopt especially in dealing with the harmful effects of inequity.

Part II
Specific effects of COVID-19

4 COVID-19 and globalisation

The reconstitution of the global world

This chapter discusses the relationship between the coronavirus disease-19 (COVID-19) pandemic and globalisation. It looks at past pandemics and traces through what we have learned about these and the coronavirus catastrophe and whether this increased knowledge will bring about a better world. One aspect is globalisation's effects on the onset and development of COVID-19. Some writers maintain that globalisation, through the proliferation of urbanisation, of international trade and opening of national borders has been behind the transmission of the virus. Coronavirus has also had substantial effects on globalisation. Some have argued that it has ranged from 'bending but not breaking,' to entering a period of 'de-globalisation.' There are parallels between making the challenges of the coronavirus and meeting the challenges of climate change. Globalisation will not be the same post-pandemic and some writers argue it may never return to pre-pandemic levels. Effects of COVID-19 on employment and the labour process are also discussed.

Background on pandemics

Marital and Barzani (2020) describe four pandemics that have occurred over the past 130 years. An H2N2 virus that started in 1889 in Turkestan and spread to Berlin and Paris and finally the US, Hong Kong and Japan. It had three waves until 1892. In 1918, the Spanish Flu started in Kansas (US) and spread by April through Europe (and to Asia). The first wave disappeared in the US but had already spread. The second wave occurred in Switzerland and most cities in the world had experienced it by October 1918. The third wave spread in early 1919. Ten per cent who contracted the flu died and deaths were assessed at 1.9–5.5 per cent of the world's population (estimated to be between 34.4 million and 100 million cases). In 1957 'Asian flu,' H2N2, began in China, became an epidemic in Hong Kong and then came to Japan. It spread throughout the world. In 1958 there was a second wave (20,000 deaths) and a third wave in 1960 (26,000 deaths). In 1968, H3N2 virus started in Hong Kong and reached Japan, the US and Britain. There were two waves. It was estimated in the US 34,000 people died compared to a baseline

DOI: 10.4324/9781003449423-6

mortality for seasonal influenza of 20,000. This was 'the mildest of the four pandemics' (Marital and Barzani 2020).

Before the COVID-19 pandemic there had been pressures on the growth of globalisation. While it may appear that it had led to unrestricted growth there had been factors such as Brexit (where Britain left the European Union in 2016) with its refocussing on local rather than global issues (MacRae et al. 2021). In addition, the US had Donald Trump as President with his claim that the future was in putting America first. There had also been the growth of populist parties in countries such as Hungary and Austria (note Peterson 2021a). These formed some of the backdrop before late 2019. The emergence of the pandemic was to affect almost everything globally.

COVID-19: What is happening to globalisation?

'The pandemic has prompted a new wave of globalisation obituaries, but the latest data and forecasts imply that leaders should plan for, and shape, a world where both globalisation and anti-globalisation pressures remain enduring features of the business environment' (Altman 2020, 1). The crisis, he maintains, caused the greatest roll back of 'international flows' we have seen. Damage done to international travel, in contrast with a steadier growth pattern, affected tourism, which provides more than the automobile industry to global output. International higher education also suffered immense slowdowns.

Many countries adopted an international diversification policy related to supply chains. COVID-19 led to the expansion of state power, and pandemic control led to competition between ideologies. New technologies rapidly advanced with the pandemic. These included robots, e-commerce and videoconferencing. Many initiatives resulting from COVID-19 could further globalisation. International travel spreads infection, so public opinion may have been against increasing globalisation based on more international travel and further opening of borders. Altman (2020) refers to globalisation under COVID-19 as a 'bend, but not break' crisis.

A far-reaching effect of COVID-19 is that it is the 'epitome of globalisation,' disrespecting borders. It may bring about the greatest 'reversal of globalisation' for decades (Toulan 2020). The practice of using low-cost countries for supplies is challenged by the growth and development of automation and robotics in more expensive regions. Countries such as South Korea which have high rates of automation weathered COVID-19 better than most. There is a widespread belief that there is too much dependence on other countries and this dependence on 'global value chains' represents a grave danger (Thangavel, Pathak and Chandra 2021).

'As horrible as the coronavirus is, several analysts suggest that it might be an opportunity to correct a global economy that ravages the environment and spurs massive income inequality' (Goffman 2020, 48). It may be possible, with the required will, to shift from materialism which is a short-term goal towards a socially beneficial approach. He (2020) argues we might develop physical movements that slow down the spread of pathogens and have beneficial environmental impacts of reduced air traffic. Goffman (2020) argues that we need *glocalisation*, that is an awareness of the environment and 'economic equity.' Based on an analysis of drivers behind the COVID pandemic Jeanne et al. (2022) argue that the 'geography of economic relations' and globalisation were mostly behind the virus spread across the globe.

In a study of the extent to which COVID-19 affected globalisation across several nations Zhang et al. (2023a) found the global average level of globalisation is anticipated to decrease between 2017 and 2025. The decrease accounting for COVID-19 is expected to be –4.76 per cent in 2025. While there is a downward trend, largely due to economic considerations, it is not as large as has been predicted. There was a positive impact of COVID-19 on globalisation in the US, Australia, Japan, India, Russia, Brazil and Togo. However, in the UK, Egypt, China, Switzerland, Qatar, China and Gabon globalisation was anticipated to decrease.

Business supply chains were disrupted during the pandemic (The Conversation 2023).Many companies had very long international supply chains. Three changes occurred. Firstly, they relocated suppliers closer to home. Secondly, they made greater investments in technology. Thirdly, they moved to carry more inventory, 'just in case' supplies ran out. In this sense planning for post-virus times resulted in a reduction of globalised activity.

A sustainable society in the future needs to confront the problems brought about by neoliberalism. Climate change and COVID-19 have in common their disregard for 'geopolitical' boundaries, and both thrived under globalisation of the 1990s (Goffman 2020). The mechanics of free trade and the incessant focus on economic growth ignored the rights of labour, with underemployment and precarious work increasing. It also largely ignored environment.

More than three years since the pandemic cast a 'shadow' over transnationalism and globalisation fundamental changes took place. New forms of capital flows, labour, social and political and cultural arrangements as well as communication technologies and platforms have resulted from disrupted global networks. Technological platforms such as Zoom and Teams have 'democratised communication.' Beaverstock et al. (2023) maintain these changes have been challenging to states and cities and to modes of governance as they have involved crossing borders. Research foci have changed to include 'transnational social sciences perspectives; networks, flows, connections, and disconnections; human agency and 'globalisation from below'; and the future of globalisation and transnationalism' (Beaverstock et al. 2023, 9). Global inequality has increased, and populism is a force. Debate about whether we have entered a period of deglobalisation continues. Post Trumpism and Brexit there is an ongoing discussion on border protection. In Australia under a conservative government border protection was a catch cry and the treatment of 'illegal immigrants' was dreadful.

Based on a series of interviews, Mathews (2023) shows how broker nego-tiations in the informal economy between Chinese suppliers and African cus-tomers have been affected by the internet expansion and COVID-19. Much of this trade is illegal and relies on bribery. He refers to this as low-end globalisation. Informal cross-border trade relies on face-to-face communica-tion, but internet growth and restrictions imposed by coronavirus have af-fected this. Mathews (2023) maintains much trade is informal and China has been the main global source of informal trade of manufactured goods. The internet has meant that African customers know the correct prices for goods, reducing bribery, and COVID-19 has meant that shipping costs increased.

Socio-political aspects of COVID-19

The pandemic has shown how the study of globalisation in the future needs to look at the operation and structure of power. How does economic inter-dependence shape identities, create contentious politics and change political authority? Writers have evaded the implications of how culture and power and transnational political authority operate. Political economy perspectives should deal with the 'big picture.' McNamara and Newman (2020) point out that basic assumptions begin with markets as constructions of social interac-tions. COVID-19 is the most recent 'shock' to globalisation. Future research needs to consider gender, race and ethnicity, class and sexual identities as responses to global markets. Globalisation as we know it is formed by 'politi-cal authority' that does not reflect traditional state control or market domi-nation over politics. 'Economic integration is creating new forms of political authority and creating links between other entities that exist outside of the state. As these sites of contention shift, so too do global politics' (McNamara and Newman 2020, E66).

Urban population density is linked to the virus spread. Barak, Sommer and Mualam (2021) analyse the effects of urban density on COVID-19. Cit-ies have particular social, political, spatial and affective structures. Cities dif-fer from each other based on their political context. This affected compliance with coronavirus regulations. In a study of Israel where 90 per cent of the population live in cities the co-workers claim that there were 'socio-urban' differences in the way the virus manifested. There are cities characterised by different ethnic and religious affiliations and heterogeneity. Where edicts for mitigating the virus (such as quarantining, lockdown) were used each city in their study had their own distinctive way of responding, making the im-pact of measures on infection rates uneven. Where there was a lack of trust in government, regulations were less effective. This was also the case when alienation was high.

In parts of Europe vaccine uptake for COVID-19 was lower than antici-pated (Zimmermann et al. 2023a). In Europe vaccination was voluntary but some countries required it for specific groups such as health professionals. However, there were restrictions for those unvaccinated, such as at border crossings. With vaccination there are individual, social and socio-political factors that come to play. That is there are pre-existing attitudes for and against vaccination; trust in government equating to confidence to vaccinate; a lack of trust in scientists and science related to hesitancy; and distrust in politics and related institutions predicts belief in conspiracy theories. Further, hesitancy is related to consuming greater amounts of information about COVID-19 than those who refuse vaccination. An additional impact on vaccination choice is through family, friends, work and even casual acquaintances, and when there were concerns about the safety and effectiveness of vaccines. Further a lack of access to vaccination facilities can inhibit their use, and public debate about vaccine mandates can reduce the choice to vaccinate.

Zimmermann et al. (2023a) argue that in general Europeans had 'different shades of doubt' on vaccination. Attitudes to vaccination depended on people's social and community context and were in a 'broader socio-political context.' Where attitudes and experiences of vaccination changed it was due to experience or new information, influence from the social environment or aspects of vaccination programmes that affected technical/logistic factors as well as social context. Debates on vaccines are highly politicised and decisions to vaccinate are not only personal, based on trust, but political and a 'judgement' on governance. Deciding not to vaccinate may be due to dissatisfaction with political leaders. Leadership on vaccination needs to account for personal experience, beyond technical and scientific data, much of which is presented as metrics. A social divide is to be avoided. For booster vaccinations there needs to be regular communication to ensure maintaining and developing public trust.

Mansouri (2020) argues that eliminating global threats requires 'transnational solidarity' and equitable capacity building. Solidarity between nations and intercultural dialogue is beneficial. Also, 'utopian, worldly and ethical approaches' can be constructive. That is, they can bring about safety, sustainability and well-being for the planet.

Globalisation and the pandemic

Shrestha et al. (2020) argue that globalisation is at the base of how many earn their living but is also the way in which pathogens spread across the world. Three aspects of globalisation are: the mobility of people, the economic sphere through workforces including supply chains, and through healthcare systems based on global health. These are indicators of the pandemic creating unparalleled burdens. 'Over the years, globalisation has amplified global disease transmission and has had significant economic implications. The close integration of the economy in modern times has, therefore, emerged as an essential mechanism of disease transmission' (Shrestha et al. 2020, 2).

It is important to investigate just how the relationship between globalisation and the pandemic plays out. There was research on the relationship in 150 countries between extent of globalisation and fatalities attributed to COVID-19. Using regression analysis Farzanagan, Feizi and Gholipor (2021) identified that where there was greater socio-economic globalisation there was a higher level of case fatality rates. This was evident after controlling for factors such as economic development, healthcare costs and capacity.

Alcalde and Escribano (2020) report on conjecture about whether there is a current period of de-globalisation. Looking firstly on the effects of globalisation on virus spread, the bubonic plague of the 14th century had devastating effects, caused by the trade routes of the Silk Roads. Later conquistadors encouraged increased globalisation and the spread of pathogens to the New World. Both World Wars had globalising impacts as colonial ties diminished. Despite COVID-19 Alcalde and Escribano (2020) argue that globalisation will continue its push, and notions of de-globalisation will be brushed aside. However, Demena, van Bergeijk and Afesorgbor (2022) argue despite global interconnectedness behind the spread of the virus, the pandemic also represents an aspect of de-globalisation. International cooperation was breaking down with a lack of support for neighbouring countries, for example with protective medical equipment and vaccines.

Gouzoulis and Galanis (2021) raise the issue of financialisaton and how it can affect COVID-19 in relation to physical distancing. Poorer communities house people and provide workers with smaller lodgings and workplaces where pathogens can more easily spread. Precarious workers in poorer economies were less likely to have suitable accommodation as a protection from infection and were more likely to spread infection if they worked in two or more workplaces. In addition, for some of the people with pension payments not adequately funding retirement, many in this most vulnerable age group for infection had to go back into the workforce and risk infection.

Chile has suffered through COVID-19. In the first half of 2020 up to two million jobs were lost (one-third of the workforce). Egana-delSol, Cruz and Micco (2022) claim that coronavirus had a very strong impact on developing countries as they have large informal sectors and a poor social safety, and financial markets are not robust. In developed countries labour markets have been bolstered by artificial intelligence (AI), computing developments, robotics and digitisation. In developing economies automation has increased employment in some areas and decreased it in others. However, those at risk of automation have had the greatest job loss (about 7% less employment between the end of 2019 and March/April 2021). In Chile, informal workers were affected at three times the rate of those in the formal sector.

The term social distancing has often been used to refer to keeping at a safe distance from others during the virus. The use of the term physical distancing is correct. In a sociocultural sense the idea of social distancing is a misnomer, according to Mansouri (2020).What is meant by social distancing is physical distancing. Social distancing means to establish social and cultural barriers, and that is not meant when the term social distancing is used to mitigate COVID-19 spread.

As discussed earlier globalisation, through the proliferation of urbanisation, international trade and the opening of national borders has been a breeding ground for virus transmission. With COVID-19 there have been the shortening of supply chains and difficulty in protecting workers, particularly for frontline health and mobile workers. These aspects have led to increased risk and hardship.

Social construction in the pandemic

There is an argument that COVID-19 and climate change are two aspects of a 'hegemonic social representation' of survival, shared with democracy, nature and science. Magioglou and Coen (2021) claim this is a useful tool for conceptualising changes in individual and group thought and dynamics. It helps to navigate meanings in competing situations of constructions related to survival. It can also help in action related to climate change.

Since the start of the pandemic old age has been made vulnerable by the media highlighting it as risky (Gallistl et al. 2023). This represents what gerontologists have called ageism. In a qualitative study the researchers found that for older people age was characterised by 'not doing,' particularly not everyday routines. This is what makes them feel vulnerable. As a societal response, activity represents positive ageing, but during COVID-19 there were not a lot of opportunities for maintaining being active.

Abeysinghe et al. (2022) argue that the 'lay construction of risk' affects the delivery of public health and is behind social responses to COVID-19. In Jakarta (Indonesia) digital diaries were used over five weeks early in the pandemic to record the experiences of a small sub-set of the population on risk production. The construction of risk was related to physical distancing and feeling confused about government actions. The 'ignorant imagined other' was how people see themselves related to being at risk from 'unknowledgeable others.' This represented risk in a social location against an imagined other in response to public health policy and activities.

In a study of China and India, Hossain, Shi and Jahan (2023) explain governance, communication and construction of risk related to COVID-19. Due to policy narratives and communication, there is a social construction of public perception. They (2023) argue the setting of culture and risk narratives strongly affect crisis management. Previous studies have not included socio-political, governance and leadership styles in constructing risk through public perception. China used health diplomacy as a tool in relation to coronavirus. It has had more success than India in creating narratives of the social construction of risk.

Sandhu and Barn (2022) studied urban middle class children (aged 16–17 years) in India during the coronavirus lockdown. Indian children's use of digital technologies is based on gender, class and location. There are discrepancies between 'media-poor' and 'media rich' childhoods. Lockdown exposed 'media-rich' children to certain risks and the young people looked for digital opportunities in the social construction of the self. Sandhu and Barn (2022) looked at how engaging with technology helped shape young people's well-being. Young people dealt with failures of networks, online class demands and their mental health and relationships. During times of crisis the social construction of the self for these young people developed using digital technology. In India it depends on social structure and reproducing social inequality.

The context of COVID-19

COVID-19 emerged as a global crisis at a time when neoliberal globalisation was at its peak. This was a time when countries were dependent on ever increasing supply chains and extensive trade. In Chapter 3 (see Navarro [2020] neoliberal policies are discussed as the antithesis of effective ways of dealing with the pandemic. Neoliberal policies have created precarious work and consequent mental health problems for groups of workers including nurses (Rezio et al. 2022).

Altman and Bastian (2022) have argued that the Russian invasion of Ukraine has raised concerns that the end of globalisation is near, much in the same way that the onset of the COVID pandemic did. Yet 'cross-border flows' between countries have reoccurred since the initial stages of the pandemic. Similarly, the war will cause some reduction of global activity affecting food supplies including sanctions but will not lead to the demise of international business flows. However, there will be restrictions.

The pandemic of 1918, Hong Kong flu in the 1970s and the SARS pandemic have all had effects on societies. The 1918 pandemic led to reduced education, diminished socio-economic status and an increase in disabilities. Pandemics can lead to reduced workforce participation and school absenteeism. They have also led to reduced economic and human capital. The COVID-19 pandemic has changed the world. It devastated economies worldwide and dramatically affected health (Shrestha et al. 2020). There was a reduction in mobility including reduced air and sea travel, as well as trade and travel restrictions. Major industries have been upset including events cancellations, limitations on workforces, and some workers having to engage in dangerous practices (see Neis et al. 2021 on truckers, seafarers, meat process workers and in the mobile labour force). In addition, there have been drastic effects on healthcare capacity, food and agriculture, including limiting production and supply chains. The ten most vulnerable countries to coronavirus reported by Shrestha et al. (2020) were Brazil, India, US, Russia, South Africa, Chile, Mexico, Iran, Peru and Pakistan.

Overpopulated cities and the removal of borders globally were prerequisites for a pandemic. A shift to more sustainable models away from mass consumption and mass production is required. A major issue is that the systems remaining in countries such as Brazil and the US prioritised economics over preventing infection. The problem with the epidemic is the creation of vulnerable economic and social systems (Yoshimitsu 2020).

Tabbush (2021) argues that economically COVID-19 has had a greater impact on women with 435 million globally in extreme poverty. She predicts there will be 118 women compared to 100 men in poverty globally because of the virus. Lewis (2020) reports that in many countries there has been increased workload for women as they have had to shoulder more of the unpaid childcare when schools have closed.

The 'blame game' between the US and China is a facet of state responses during coronavirus (Jaworsky and Qiaoan 2021). They report a rise in nationalism during the pandemic that has intensified by the US claiming China to be the cause of the pandemic. (The US under President Donald Trump focussed on Wuhan as the source of the pandemic and raised the issue of compensation). The researchers (2021) use a cultural sociological approach into the meaning of the 'narrative battle' between the two countries. The relationship between the two superpowers was the most important during the pandemic.

The rise of nationalism threatened globalisation, meaning that governments and business communities needed to establish new ways of operating (Yaya, Otu and Labonté 2020). An outcome of nationalism and conflicting aspects of globalisation has been labelled 'slowbalisation,' evidenced by declining foreign investment and trade. They argue that COVID-19 bought about uncertainty and fear. Globalisation over several decades has now faced major threats. Yaya et al. (2020) maintain Africa's disrupted supply chains have led to unemployment and poverty. Their reliance on gas and oil has been too great and led to vulnerability. Also, lockdowns may not have been a best way of dealing with the pandemic in Africa. Globalisation although has been beneficial to some African countries. COVID-19 disrupted Africa's 'global supply chains' seeing oil prices falling and a lesser demand for other African products. This posed a threat economically (Yaya et al. 2020). Before COVID-19 Africa faced deteriorating healthcare facilities and structure. Ozili (2020) reports that 65 per cent of their healthcare expenditure is out of pocket, compared to less in many other regions. COVID-19 has affected African regions most severely.

McCausland (2020) argues that some positives to emerge from COVID-19 included that scientists globally have been mobilised in mostly worldwide cooperation. In addition, the World Health Organisation (WHO) facilitated international efforts to develop vaccines, strengthening the sharing of information. The pandemic has highlighted the need for enhanced emergency services. Assefa et al. (2022) argue that all countries were at risk. National strategies are required to improve the management of public health emergencies, to develop sufficient public health capacity and to address social and economic imbalance. They maintain primary health methods, a holistic government, and an appropriate societal process could achieve this.

For some, COVID-19 is seen as reducing globalisation, while to others globalisation will remain based on established principles. The virus uncovers globalised trends that are already in operation, focussing on re-shaping identities, power relations and some newer contentious politics. 'We see .... transformational dynamics at work in at least four areas: inequality within and across societies, new forms of economic statecraft, existential ecological threats, and the trajectory of the digital revolution' (McNamara and Newman 2020, E60).

The pandemic, globalisation and the labour process

Dorflinger, Valeria and Vallas (2021) focus on the labour process of logistic workers in addressing their contribution to the smooth flowing of global capitalism. In ports delivery workers have a large latent power to disrupt the flow of goods, but in the main they have not used that power. 'What mechanisms account for capital's ability to limit logistics workers' structural power? Put differently, how is class dominance maintained within the logistics industry's many ports, warehouses, and shipping networks?' (Dorflinger et al. 2021, 112). Their study, conducted until mid-2019, did not include specific effects of the coronavirus since, but given that supply chains are shorter in most countries because of COVID-19, it is expected that the labour process has significantly changed. It has especially been the case in African countries.

There are challenges based on labour process analysis of working from home initiated by coronavirus (Bromfield 2022). Disadvantages include increases in unpaid work, being constantly available and downloading costs of production. There are certain advantages including increased autonomy. Work from home will continue but its downside is fewer social relations. Manokha (2020) argues that working from home or remotely in western nations was welcomed by many and telework is seen as potentially the norm for many. He argues that normalising telework and blurring home/work divisions, as well as collapsing divisions between professional/private life, have come about because of work undertaken during COVID-19.

The effect of the coronavirus on labour has been huge. The class struggle during neoliberalism characterises disputes of distribution in capitalism, and this can disregard needing to challenge capital in terms of property and production relations. During COVID-19 household incomes of workers, which are traditionally the 'site of redistributive struggle,' are used more as supportive income streams as a basis of asset accumulation by the propertied class (Heenan and Sturman 2020).

'Health workers labouring during conditions of crisis .... might be thought of as being immune to injury or illness because their job is to heal the sick and injured. They are very vulnerable because they commonly prioritise their patients' needs above their own' (Harrell, Selvaraj and Edgar 2020, 1). In a review of the literature the co-workers outline the effects of coronavirus and other disasters on health workers. These include problems in supply lines resulting in deficiencies – long hours of work including staff shortages and the transmission of infections. Also there have been physical and mental fatigue and post-traumatic stress disorder (PTSD). Those with adaptability and resilience and who have had structured training were less exposed to risk.

Burnout, poor job satisfaction and health issues have accompanied emotional labour (Gamage 2023) and intensified during the pandemic. More resources, training and help with family issues, were needed by healthcare personnel in the wake of mental health issues experienced during the virus. Gamage (2023) argued that human resource management is needed to provide strategies and resources to help frontline employees to deal with emotionally challenging and extreme work conditions. Organisations needed to better understand the cognitive aspects of workers involved in this field of work. There can be greater support for well-being, engagement and effective functioning. Organisations need to provide resources for line managers. These changes will focus more attention on job demands and resources. The pandemic may give a way of better understanding the consequences of emotional work.

The growth of telework is likely to persist after the coronavirus crisis as the growth in 24/7 work continues. One caution offered by Manokha (2020) is there is a growth of employee surveillance at home with digital means in private homes normalising surveillance in personal space. There is a new type of alienation with telework, from the worker's home. When at home they are under the penetrating gaze of their employer into their 'private space' while working in the context of relaxing and living their home-based life. Separate work and home time occurred especially in the period following the second World War. However, in what Manokha refers to as 'flexible capitalism' in the modern era the juncture between labour and rest has been disrupted. That is, as he refers to Marx (1976), capitalist production looks to appropriating labour through the whole of 24 hours. Through modern times and working at home arrangements the juncture between work and rest is dissipating.

Conclusion

In academic and non-academic literature COVID-19 has been shown to have had a huge effect on globalisation. This has affected international travel, shortened supply chains, slowed international education and radically affected the movements and interactions of people across the globe. For some this heralded a slowdown or even finish of globalisation, while others maintain that globalisation is resilient enough to bend, rather than break. COVID-19 has had an enormous impact on employment and on the way we work, with some work regarded as essential, but there have been large groups unemployed.

The move to working from home that applies to many industries has positive and negative aspects. Issues such as home and work balance have become blurred as many women have taken on increased unpaid domestic care where children are involved. Some researchers have argued that home-based employees experience increased alienation. Employment post-pandemic may not be the same as prior to the virus. Some labour is likely now to be home based or at least hybrid, and traditional divisions between women's and men's labour are likely to be intensified, including domestic unpaid labour.

5 The impact of COVID-19 on national and global health and safety at work (OHS)

There are several approaches to occupational health and safety (OHS), some highlighting socio-political perspectives embodied in political economy approaches, some focussing on economic factors, and some with broader foci on national and global issues. One aspect of OHS over the recent past has been globalised organisations employing increasing numbers of precarious workers. The growth in precarity during globalisation has been extensive, and this has replaced post World War 2 stability in employment, which saw permanent full-time work gradually subside. Labour markets are now characterised by underemployment and less secure work. In terms of OHS risk, Europe has reported stress as the second most prevalent occupational illness and injury (ILO 2020a) and in several OECD countries it has been extensive together with claims of bullying and harassment.

This chapter begins by looking at pressures bought to bear in the workplace due to the pandemic. Further it examines OHS in relation to coronavirus disease-19 (COVID-19) and the nature of that relationship. The impact on OHS of coronavirus in several different countries is further discussed as well as the effects of the pandemic on unemployment and what this means for health.

Introduction

The advent of the pandemic bought with it a plethora of challenges to labour markets and OHS internationally. Mobile workers have been strongly affected by COVID-19 (Neis et al. 2021). Many of these experienced high risks of infection and endured poor and cramped living conditions. In addition, frontline health workers were up to three times more likely to be infected by the virus than other workers. In many cases there had been an under supply of personal protective equipment (PPE). Post-traumatic stress disorder has also been reported amongst many frontline health workers in countries hardest hit by the pandemic such as in Italy.

In addition to infection, over time a recession may be an outcome with associated effects on employment, but this has been confined to selected countries. By late 2023 many developed countries have attempted to guard

DOI: 10.4324/9781003449423-7

against a post-pandemic recession. Leading up to this time some banks in the US and in Europe collapsed. OHS regulation can have an important part to play giving workers and organisations advice about safe employment to help deal with the health consequences of a possible recession (Godderis and Luyten 2020). Recession can have mixed effects on mortality and morbidity, with differing outcomes depending on socio-economic group. COVID-19, impact of lockdowns and the threat of recessions might expand health inequalities. 'A striking finding from health research on recessions is that a recession typically has bigger impact on the health of vulnerable, disadvantaged groups, lowest-paid employees, migrant workers and those working in the informal economy' (Godderis and Luyten 2020, 511).

OHS and COVID-19 effects

COVID-19 has affected nearly every type of work. OHS frontiers were pushed when virus outbreaks were placing workers, families and whole regions at risk. As well as possible infection, workers had to deal with new ways of working to reduce infection spread. Sustaining morale of workers at home proved a major management issue and increases in computer vision syndrome occurred with long hours spent working in front of screens. There were new OHS guidelines to alleviate many of these problems (Ramos et al. 2022).

'Health workers may be exposed to occupational hazards that put them at risk of disease, injury and even death in the context of the virus response .... includ(ing) (a) occupational infections with COVID-19; (b) skin disorders and heat stress from prolonged use of PPE; (c) exposures to toxins because of increased use of disinfectants; (d) psychological distress; (e) chronic fatigue; and (f) stigma, discrimination, physical and psychological violence and harassment' (WHO 2021a, 2). World Health Organization (WHO) outlines measures protecting OHS of health workers and focussed on rights, responsibilities and duties of OHS in relation to the virus.

De Oliveira et al. (2022) present an analysis of the WHO's directives on OHS in the light of COVID-19. WHO practices reduced by half the effects of COVID-19 on performance, but only negligibly addressed the negative effects on health and safety leading to increased absenteeism. The pandemic has harmed physical and mental health and resistance, affecting employees' safety. WHO developed OHS arrangements including work area redesign to allow the maintenance of physical distance, the allocation of 'new work shifts,' PPE using respirators and masks, the measurement of temperature, as well as hand hygiene and equipment for disinfecting possibly contaminated surfaces (De Oliveira et al. 2022). A significant gain on organisational performance was through minimising the transmission of COVID-19. Benefits were through acting on OHS using education, information and communication to workers.

COVID-19 disrupted economies, public health systems and medical-care. It also reshaped working futures. The structure of work has changed with large effects on companies and the health and well-being of workers. Employers, government and public health organisations, trade unions and professional associations have struggled with economic objectives at the same time as keeping employees healthy and safe (Peters et al. 2022). The virus has bought about changes in economic, social and political environments influencing labour patterns. In some countries the response to the pandemic has been effective, and in several jurisdictions, the outcomes of COVID-19 policies have led to trust in government.

In a qualitative study spanning ten countries Gold, Hughes and Thomas (2021) report on an expanded role for OHS which included resilience and well-being, business continuity and assessing and responding to risks during COVID-19. The pandemic had three consequences, namely post-traumatic stress disorder, stress and burnout. According to Dubey et al. (2020), there has been increased job insecurity. Management had a greater responsibility to balance safety, production and profit and to reduce work-related stress due to COVID-19. One of the crucial effects of adopting OHS procedures was absenteeism reduction due to contamination. Re-establishing work locations (1.5-m spacing) reduced absenteeism through infection, and medical leave allowed a more secure recovery time at home. More changing rooms, toilets and washbasins (including sanitisers) in workplaces were also critical, as were improvements in ventilation. However even while having an N 95 mask, effective on-the-job training, a risk management programme and work safety organisation, negative impacts on safety still occurred. For example, PPE standards have not been sufficient in health and hospitality services. Poorer workers were disadvantaged. There had been difficulties experienced in relation to WHO guidelines on physical distancing including reorganising tables/benches for 1.5-m spacing, more shifts and rotations of work, mandatory mask wearing at work, more washbasins, bathrooms and gel for hand hygiene, water and soap. These measures were used before return-to-work services in Spain. Companies were needing to encourage the trust of their employees.

In several essential jobs which involved facing the public, for example in supermarkets, correctional facilities and healthcare, workers dealt with increased work demand and high COVID-19 risk. In food industries, warehousing and manufacture these essential jobs may have been in crowded locations without adequate ventilation and with high risk of infection (Peters et al. 2022). Workers able to transition to working from home were more likely to be urban, with higher incomes and more stability.

Changing labour patterns

Automation of jobs has increased due to COVID-19. Peters et al. (2022) argue that worldwide workers in non-standard jobs such as gig, contract and agency-based work have increased since 2008. This is more so due to COVID-19. The consequent increase in flexibility for employers can lead to more injury, less security and more health risks. This is so even where the flexibility suits some employees. Overall, indigenous workers and those from ethnic and race minority and immigrant workers have been affected more. Much of this work is for low wages in essential jobs which have an elevated risk of infection. Canada and the UK are just two countries where employees with disabilities faced substantial disadvantage in relation to COVID-related 'work accommodations' (Peters et al. 2022).

Rivera-Cuadrado (2023) maintains a defining feature of healthcare in the pandemic was occupational risk. Frontline workers risked their health and safety to sustain the health system. They had raised infection rates, lost lives, had burnout and trauma. Understanding their risk experience will help with any future pandemics. The researcher (2023) argues for qualitative methods to better understand practitioner risk. There were three concerns for the health workers: first working in the COVID-19 context required adaptation and regarding their bodies as possibly hazardous; second there were limitations of protective measures putting them at odds with patient care; and third managing the virus meant dealing with known and unknown risks. There were two aspects of risk. They came from occupational, not medical factors, and they had direct exposure to infected patients.

A socio-political perspective shows how labour patterns have affected organisations and workers (note Peterson 2021c). As COVID-19 progressed several organisations reduced their activities on well-being and communication in the workplace. Healthcare, food, retail and education, for example, have redesigned work to reduce exposure to the virus: many other benefits may flow on. The coronavirus has had extended effects on organisations, employees and the global future of work. Impacts remain uncertain. The relationship between COVID-19 and population health has come to the fore as has employee metal health and well-being. Peters et al. (2022) argue that these have extended the scope of OHS which prior to COVID centred on risk of injury and disease. The focus has turned to the positive effects of work on the 'thriving in life' of workers.

An overall integrated framework for keeping workers safe during COVID-19 was proposed by Dennerlein et al. (2020). They state that health, safety and well-being of essential workers, particularly those who are in contact with the public, was severely impacted by the virus. This had been even during stay-at-home mandates. Interactions can be stressful when not knowing the 'infection statuses' of others. Public health responses affected how people interact and live. These changes have been very stressful. COVID-19 means that in the workplace constructive infection control is required to reduce harmful exposure and these include an increase of ventilation and high-quality air filters. Physical barriers between customers and workers were required as well as physical distancing. Handwashing facilities were needed, as well as PPE. In addition, increasing psychological pressures on essential employees can be met by having appropriate working conditions. Workers might have their well-being threatened due to virus exposure, increased pace and demands of work and problems in relation to home and work balance (such as with childcare). Flexible breaks, using participative approaches, accurate communication and a social environment that is supportive all helped with the extra demands on employees (Dennerlein et al. 2020).

Coronavirus and OHS across different countries

As a result of COVID-19 the way work is carried out has changed. It has affected worker/employer relations. Some people could work from home creating a 'new normal,' while others, often in more physical work, were working longer, some in compromised workplaces (Orvitz 2021). For many employees their jobs have become harder and more stressful. The UK Household Longitudinal Study found mental distress grew by 8.1 per cent in April 2020, from 2017/19 figures. The researcher (2021) argues that for many employees, mental health support was needed.

In the US more than 60 per cent of people in the same job as they were before the onset of COVID-19 said they were as satisfied with their job now as before. Their security and productivity had not changed (Parker, Horowitz and Minkin 2020). Of those now working from home or hybrid (home and workplace but not before coronavirus), almost half say they can choose to work flexible hours, more so than those who previously also worked from home or hybrid (only 14% could choose hours worked). Also, 38 per cent of those newly working from home said balancing home and work responsibilities was easier, but 65 per cent felt less connection now with their co-workers. Also, in the US Leppert (2023) reports that by 2023 young workers now were less likely to report higher job satisfaction compared to older workers with 85 per cent somewhat satisfied overall with their job.

As a background to resources which affect COVID-19 deaths, an analysis of healthcare system indicators and European mortality due to coronavirus was carried out by Mattiuzzi, Lippi and Henry (2021). The death rate due to COVID-19 in EU countries was negatively related to health facilities and resources (hospitals, nurses and doctors). Positive relationships existed with acute bed occupancy, and the proportion of 65 years and older, weight and cancer. These factors mainly explained EU COVID-19 deaths. Healthcare expenditure and hospital beds were not related to the death rate.

To cope with the pandemic OHS has had to adjust. 'OHS are a unique type of business and are in a unique position to undergo change to manage their services during a pandemic which pose a major risk to healthcare workers' (Ranka, Quigley and Hussain 2020, 359). A cross-sectional survey was completed by 62 OHS practitioners from the UK in the initial stages of COVID-19. Fifty-four per cent had changed the way they worked, and 51 per cent offered out-of-hours and weekend services. Sixty per cent offered no vaccination service, and 54 per cent of OHS services offered reviews of active

Occupational Dermatitis cases and needle stick injuries. Fifty-six per cent offered a COVID-19 telephone helpline (45% of OHS service had a separate COVID-19 e-mail inbox to manage queries).

Health and Safety Executive (HSE 2022)) has stated that in Great Britain a public health body may declare an outbreak at any time in a workplace. In the later stages of the coronavirus in 2022 HSE stated that guidance on coronavirus for workplaces would be replaced by public health advice. They no longer required businesses to account for COVID-19 in their risk assessment.

The US faced a major worker health and safety crisis with the pandemic. Many employees were at risk of infection from the virus, particularly those in healthcare and performing 'essential' jobs. In the US by law employers must provide a workplace without major hazards. Michaels and Wagner (2020) maintain enforcing the law is the role of the Occupational Safety and Health Administration (OSHA) and the government had not fully used its safety authority to stem the tide of COVID-19. All workers needed protection, and those unprotected would spread the virus in their homes and communities, affecting mortality, morbidity and the economy. The researchers (2020) claim OSHA did not fulfilled its responsibilities. If employers were mandated by government to implement these regulations and have them enforced it could have bought about an adequate solution to coronavirus effects.

Watterson (2020) argued that the UK government was 'blinkered' by Brexit, and this had underwritten government cuts affecting workers and reducing OHS and healthcare budgets. Some of these shortfalls due to Brexit have been discussed by MacRae et al. (2021). Early into COVID-19 there were missed opportunities by OHS and public health organisations, government and their advisors who disregarded coronavirus warning signs. This led to greater mortality from the virus in the UK compared to Europe. Needing to have effective OHS measures quickly became evident in the initial stages. Chinese research showed transmission of the virus could occur through touching contaminated surfaces 'viral aerosolization' and contact with people who were infected but had no symptoms. Watterson (2020, 87) argues that 'knowledge of these routes should have informed decisions (in the early stages of COVID-19) in the UK about occupational health and safety precautions, availability of sanitizers, what personal protection equipment (PPE) was needed, by whom, and in what settings.' The pandemic in the UK has occurred in the context of years of health and social care and public health cuts, as well as cuts to OHS and environmental health agencies. These cuts have significantly threatened worker and patient health and safety.

Based on a survey of companies in Australia (O'Dwyer 2021) most had changed their usual way of operating in relation to the virus. The researcher referred to adaptation and not innovation. Most changes made during the earlier stages of the pandemic did not use formal Vocational and Educational Training. Training was largely informal and on the job or free from the government online. Often, existing skills of workers could be transferred without many problems. Aged care was different with some accredited training occurring, particularly in infection control. This generally was online by registered, private training organisations, self-funded or paid for by the employer.

Coronavirus contaminates workplaces leaving workers and families at risk. There were additional risks posed by new work practices implemented to curtail the virus' spread (Asada-Miyakawa 2021). Several OHS initiatives have been addressed in the Asia-Pacific region by the International Labour Organisation (ILO). Singapore has protective regulations for the vulnerable on teleworking or leave; materials on effective communication with workers and others with COVID-19 have been disseminated in India; ergonomically sound home office environment has been set up in New Zealand; problems related to trauma associated with unemployment and workplace closures have been researched in Bangladesh, and specific risks with COVID-19 faced by migrants have been addressed in Malaysia.

According to Iavicoli et al. (2021) Italy was the first western country to confront the spread of COVID-19, and they argue it was one of the hardest hit. The extent of hospital admissions due to COVID-19 and availability of intensive care beds have been a challenge to the health system. The Italian Government suspended most business activity, thereby reducing by 75 per cent the number of workers. Universities and schools were also closed. Containment measures tackled the risk of infection, which was particularly relevant to the health workforce.

In a study of frontline medical staff in China during the first year of COVID-19 job satisfaction was found to be reasonable (Yu et al. 2020). The following factors needed to be considered by management and their demands needed to be met: stronger emergency response was needed; junior staff needed operational training; and rest and sleep needs were required. Medical staff on the front line had an intensified workload, more infection risk and greater stress. These factors have the potential to affect job satisfaction. Current research on these workers was for skin conditions, anxiety, depression, mood problems, sleep issues and exercise rehabilitation (Yu et al. 2020).

The first coronavirus case reported in Poland was on March 4, 2020. In a survey of Polish employers Nowacki, Grabowska and Lakomy (2020) found that due to coronavirus 30 per cent of companies had updated occupational risk assessment and 40 per cent had revised safety instructions. A further 90 per cent had provided employees with extra PPE. In Poland the health and safety service advised employers on the safety of companies. Organisations with more than 600 employees needed to have one part-time worker performing an OHS role for each 600 employed. Organisations with 100–600 employees needed the OHS unit to have one part-time worker in that role, and for those employing up to 100 workers, the OHS role could be performed by the employer, a worker or an external specialist.

Bankova and Kutsarov (2022) examined the means through which accommodation organisations applied in responding to virus regulations established by government. Qualitative in-depth interviews were undertaken in Bulgaria. Other European countries as well as the UK were included.

The co-workers found similar health and safety procedures for COVID-19 were employed between the different countries. Chafi, Hultberg and Yams (2022) undertook a qualitative study of three Swedish public service organisations involved in healthcare and infrastructure administration. The benefits of remote and hybrid work implemented due to coronavirus were described by some as flexibility, autonomy and work-life balance. The drawbacks were social aspects and isolation.

Igarashi et al. (2022) undertook an interview-based qualitative study of the use of Occupational Physicians (OP) in Japan. Thirteen OPs were selected for the study. At work, due to the virus there were health conditions, musculoskeletal disorders, for example coming from home-based telework and mental health issues resulting from isolation, poor support and overwork. Fatigue and stress led to mistakes and resulted in incidents. OPs are expected to support the organisation affected by COVID-19. They provided support on the direct effects of the virus by giving professional information and advising the organisation and workers in the context of the company's risk management. They also provided support on the indirect effects of coronavirus. Work systems had been implemented at times with little preparation. Therefore, OPs helped with a range of problems: these included psychosocial factors, for example stress related to work and home balance and insufficient supervisory and co-worker support; ergonomic factors, for example musculoskeletal problems from working in unsuitable environments; problems of stigma and discrimination against those infected with the virus and their families; and those who refused to vaccinate. OPs were asked to give their company information on these problems as a preventative measure.

How work was performed prior to and during COVID-19 is vastly different. The future of work is open to conjecture. Champagne, Granja and Choiniere (2023) discuss changing work arrangements in Canada. Flexible working arrangement was not effectively utilized prior to the virus. By 2023 work restrictions due to COVID-19 had been lifted, requiring workers to spend 40–60 per cent of their work time in the workplace. Further return to the workplace, particularly for public service workers, is a contentious issue. Champagne et al. (2023) suggest that a return to pre-pandemic work practices is not likely.

Developing economies

There was a cross-sectional action research study undertaken of the health workforce in South Africa. Data was collected on OHS systems in 45 hospitals to identify aspects of protection for health workers (Zungu et al. 2021). They had been at risk of infection. Reports from China suggested increased health risk of SARS-CoV-2, depended on undertaking work that entailed risk of respiratory aerosol production, working long hours and suboptimal hand hygiene. An endemic problem was a shortage of staff. They report WHO projections that by 2030 there will be a shortage of approximately 18 million health workers, with Southeast Asia and Africa the most affected. HealthWISE is a tool for identifying hazards, such as COVID-19 and undertaking control measures in lower- and middle-income countries. In terms of COVID-19 HealthWISE encouraged managers and workers to seek to 'improve SARS-CoV-2 Infection Prevention and Control (IPC) and OHS interventions.'

Sepadi and Nkosi (2022) report on OHS for street vendors, also in South Africa during COVID-19. A systematic review found the main OHS risks were due to non-enclosed vendor stalls and the regular use of open fires. The main risks were infections such as influenza and coronavirus as well as gastrointestinal diseases. These were the result of poor access to water, unsafe waste disposal arrangements and hygiene practices. Compliance with OHS regulations was therefore difficult.

Hailu et al. (2021) point out more attention is needed in African countries because of limited healthcare infrastructure. The WHO lists Ethiopia as 12th of 13 high-risk African countries (they have direct links with or a high rate of travel to China). In the initial stages of coronavirus Ethiopia did not enforce a travel ban although the virus had spread to 134 countries. After four confirmed cases, public gatherings, schools and sporting events were suspended, and soon after Ethiopian Airlines ceased flights to 30 affected countries. Hailu et al. (2021) focussed their study on the 'safety of health professionals' and their patients/clients, and modes of reducing the spread of infection in North Showa Zone, Oromia Regional State, Ethiopia. This study of 280 health professionals showed that only half reported positive OHS. Having this number with unfavourable OHS may negatively affect health professionals' lives, client health and health service outcomes. The study also identified various predictors of OHS amongst health professionals. In Ethiopia, access to soap and bleach, being able to isolate suspected cases, having 'infection prevention and control' and effective policy had a significant positive relationship to OHS practices. Where there was infection prevention and control programs in hospitals the health professionals' health and safety increased more than twofold.

Waste and sanitation workers in Bangladesh are continually exposed to hazards (Sharior et al. 2023). This risk increased during COVID-19. A qualitative study was conducted with 61 key informants where it was found that coronavirus posed severe health risks. There was poor OHS practice due to a lack of safe cleaning methods and funding. Problems included poor facilities, inadequate pay and a lack of PPE. In addition, there was little health support by the organisations, a lack of proper training and no handwashing facilities. Although the Bangladesh Labor Act (2006) focusses on the health and hygiene for all workers, these were not practised. The researchers (2023) recommend more automation and improving safety equipment.

Unemployment because of COVID-19

According to Suomi, Schofield and Butterworth (2020) unemployment rose to its highest level since the Great Depression with the onset of COVID-19. From March to April 2020 unemployment rose in the US 'from 4.4 percent to over 14.7 percent' and increased from '5.4 to 11.7 percent' in Australia. By July 2020 many countries were experiencing economic and health crises.

In Australia, a wage subsidy scheme called 'Jobkeeper' allowed employers to keep their employees in work. In Australia and the US, for example, welfare carries quite a lot of stigma, and COVID-19 bought with it several derogatory stereotypes. However, actions such as increasing welfare payments for Jobseeker (unemployment benefit) softened the harsh negative attitudes towards welfare recipients. It was clear that their lack of being in a job was not their own doing. The concept of deservedness is often applied to welfare recipients, but this 'softened' during COVID-19 (Suomi et al. 2020). Many such measures were enacted in Australia and some other countries to soften the effects of the pandemic (Munawar et al. 2021). Due to lockdown measures and the closing of borders small to medium businesses were closed and tourism suffered great losses. Universities also suffered much unemployment as the Federal Government did not offer them protective Job Keeper payments to retain their staff. In an analysis of the Australian Bureau of Census and Statistics data Churchill (2020) maintains there were gendered differences in relation to employment due to the virus. Young women had problems in gaining employment which the researcher argues rescinded some of the gains they had made in relation to work over decades.

The pandemic principally caused harm and damage to the disadvantaged. Antipova (2021) argues that there were job losses, housing difficulties, disturbance to healthcare and delays to medical treatment, culminating in premature death. Long-term effects of shocks on unemployment by the virus have been studied by Bianchi, Bianchi and Song (2021). They estimated that the COVID-19 shocks were up to five times worse than that of a regular period of unemployment, given the effects of race and gender.

The 1918 pandemic had comparatively minor economic damage compared to that associated with COVID-19 (Nga, Ramlan and Naim 2021). Pandemics have long-term consequences due to economic downturns, especially unemployment. The co-workers report on a study in Malaysia that showed professional and younger workers in particular faced hardships due to COVID-19. Apart from the airline industry in Malaysia, many others were affected. In-depth interviews of a selection of people unemployed due to the virus were carried out in Denmark by Pultz, Hansen and Jepsen (2021) and showed there were conflicts between job seeking and other demands such as family.

A study by Juranek et al. (2021) presents data on labour market effects of COVID-19 on Nordic countries. They looked at policy variations in the Nordics, between countries exposed equally to COVID-19: however, the countries responded differently. Despite having a softer lockdown, Sweden had lower unemployment than other Nordic countries in the early months of the pandemic. Developed countries with resilient health systems prior to COVID-19 were more vulnerable to the pandemic and its economic consequences (Su et al. 2021). Coronavirus affected supply chains, travel and the stability of stock markets. Globally there were disruptions to imports and exports and travel restrictions further reduced economic activity. The virus severely affected the number of working hours and unemployment, even worse than during the Global Financial Crisis. Women and younger workers have been most affected. Finally, OHS has been influenced by a worldwide shortage of workers in the healthcare industry.

Conclusion

Globally how COVID-19 affected OHS and the response of countries to providing safe and healthy work environment is a key to future work and safety arrangements. It provides a framework for responding to global threats in the future, including new pandemics, global warming/climate change and associated challenges to safety and well-being. Of particular importance is the strain put on workers who cannot work from home, and particularly those on the front lines in delivering health services to people with the virus. In many cases their health and safety had been compromised.

The world has had the threat of recession nearly four years after the onset of COVID-19. This was predicted by many researchers and commentators. Coupled with staff shortages in several areas and in particularly healthcare, government intervention is required as leaving it to neoliberalism and the market to deal with it will only result in accentuating the current lines of inequality. This will lead to more extremes of disadvantage for some groups and some nations.

6 Effects of the COVID-19 pandemic on work, technology and social relations

This chapter outlines how economies worldwide have been challenged by coronavirus disease-19 (COVID-19) and how dealing with the virus provides important lessons for effectively addressing challenges in the future. Changes in the way that work is carried out due to the onset and prevalence of the COVID pandemic are discussed. In addition, the upsurge of technology as work for many was confined to the home is outlined. Finally, consequences of COVID-19 in terms of stress, and work and home life balance are outlined and evaluated.

COVID-19: Dealing with economic issues

Several writers have discussed economic downturns due to COVID-19. In Australia as in many countries, international borders were closed which had an immediate impact on tourism and higher education for international students (Lim et al. 2021). While online teaching was embraced for some time there was severe income loss. By mid-2021 17,000 university jobs in Australia were lost. Internationally there were huge fiscal supports in advanced economies to aid domestic economic downturns. These were related to the use of lockdown measures to protect against infection.

There was large-scale financial support in many developed countries to help with local economic conditions due to the virus. The US Federal government bought about several fiscal stimulus and relief measures, being about 13 per cent of GDP. Packages (worth per cent of GDP) were implemented also in Canada (16%), Japan (21%) and Australia (14%) (Lim et al. 2021).

One of the consequences of the pandemic was an increase in unemployment, particularly for young people. Pak et al. (2020) report reduced incomes, increased unemployment and transport, manufacturing and service industry disruptions. Globally most governments had underestimated the COVID-19 risk. Given its impact is likely to be around for some time, governments needed to work towards both saving lives and preserving economic prosperity.

Based on an analysis of unemployment in Australia by Suomi, Schofield and Butterworth (2020), negative stereotypes of the unemployed were found.

DOI: 10.4324/9781003449423-8

There could be a more positive outlook towards the unemployed through extra government support. This could be a base for implementing programmes such as Universal Basic Income. In some international trials these types of programmes have demonstrated that the psychosocial profile and 'statuses' of those on welfare have been bolstered, and some of the barriers between them and the rest of society have been softened.

COVID-19 has had direct impacts on premature death as well as income, absence at work, reductions in productivity and 'negative supply shocks' with global supply chain disruptions (Pak et al. 2020). Consumers spent less due to decreased income, and many governments enacted large funding activities and increased welfare spending. Tourism, hospitality, overseas education and transport activities, however, decreased substantially.

There have been large economic impacts of the COVID-19 virus containment measures. Verschuur, Koks and Hall (2021) use data tracking on vessel activity to identify trade losses in the initial stages of the virus. China, the Middle East and Western Europe showed the greatest loss of supply chains such as automobile manufacturing and oil. Manufacturing sectors were affected most. Low-income economies and some small islands had the greatest relative trade downturns. Verschuur et al. (2021) argue that this type of data helps governments in planning economic recovery by funding the hardest hit sectors.

In a survey of 19 countries by Pew Research Centre (Silver and Connaughton 2022) many people were satisfied with their country's management of the pandemic with 68 per cent feeling their country performed well (except for Japan). Most felt COVID-19 had been divisive in their country with some shortcomings politically. Sixty-five per cent of executives surveyed by McKinsey (2021a) 18 months after the pandemic began believed their economic prospects would improve, down from six months earlier. The delta variant was one of the major concerns. Also, 49 per cent saw the pandemic as a risk to economic growth. Disruptions to supply chains, inflation and COVID-19 were the three greatest reported risks to domestic growth. The top economic risk reported (except for Latin America) was the pandemic. Respondents from developed economies saw COVID-19 as a greater threat to growth than did those from developing economies.

A short-term view in the US under COVID-19 found that unemployment increased. Negative labour market effects were greater for younger workers, the lower educated and Hispanics, meaning that COVID-19 emphasises inequities in the labour market (Beland, Broder and Wright 2020). They estimated that people working close to others were more affected, and with workers engaging in remote work less affected. The COVID-19 pandemic has bought the largest jobs crisis since the Great Depression. Inequities and poverty were to increase and impact into the future. Much needed to be done to halt the jobs crisis which may become a social crisis according to OECD (2021a). They say a more resilient labour market is needed.

Singh et al. (2021) conducted a telephone survey of the COVID effects on health and income of 2,335 people with chronic conditions in India. These were more prone to hospitalisation, intensive care and death from the virus. People had worsening hypertension and diabetes symptoms, and this was associated with difficulties in gaining medicines and job loss. Based on qualitative data most experienced distress because of job and income loss and problems in accessing health services. Those with chronic conditions, especially in rural, poor and marginalised areas had been affected financially and socially by the virus.

Bauer et al. (2020) maintain that COVID-19 created an economic as well as a public health crisis in the US. Lives have been disrupted and the hospital system reached its capacity: there had been a significant economic downturn. An unprecedented economic upheaval created demand and supply shocks. Australia had one of the best approaches to the pandemic according to O'Sullivan, Rahamathulla and Pawar (2020). Physical distancing, testing rates and financial and political stability all contributed. Dealing with inequity and vulnerable sections of community meant that social and economic recovery was most likely.

While McLaughlin (2021) reported some global economic recovery from COVID-19 in 2021 thousands of the virus variants tracked, including Delta, meant increased danger. There was also the possibility of a 'vaccine-resistant strain' to occur amongst the unvaccinated. However, in poorer countries vaccines can be scarce, offering little overall protection.

Prior to the pandemic, economies were changing. Decarbonisation and Brexit were impacting many regions. With COVID-19 came hybrid work and shutdowns which placed enormous pressures on many industries. In 2020, the global economy decreased by 4.3 per cent (Ozkan 2021). The UK had its worst recession in the recent past. OECD and World Economic Forum data showed at least Germany, South Korea, the US and Japan were expected to recover economically by the end of 2021 from pre-pandemic levels. Spain and Iceland were not expected to recover until mid-2023, and South Africa and Argentina not until late 2024 or into 2025. Ozkan (2021) argues that the strength of policy in relation to the pandemic and the vaccination programme most strongly affects economic recovery. Many poorer countries faced a long wait for vaccines, and there are significant differences in both receiving vaccines and vaccinating the population. This helped to create uneven economic consequences.

McKinsey (2021b) reported that in the US coronavirus hospitalisation rates of those immunised were comparable with rates of those hospitalised with influenza. They also report on vaccination rates across countries by September 2021. By nine months after the initial mass vaccination programme started, just 1.4 per cent of those in low-income countries had received one dose. This problem refers to the distribution and a 'strong cold-chain infrastructure' in some countries.

Structural drivers of inequity

COVID-19 emphasised the 'structural drivers of health inequities,' including precarity and harmful working conditions, large economic differences and undemocratic political activities and organisations. These have links with class, gender, ethnicity, education and other factors during coronavirus, exacerbating social susceptibilities (Paremoer et al. 2021). Precarious, adverse and exploitative work affected these sociopsychological factors for groups most exposed to the virus. Those working precariously had limited healthcare services and sick leave and could not afford adequate water, food and housing. Due to losing income and not being able to work from home they may not wish to quarantine. Slaughterhouse work for example is hazardous let alone without the virus, and the pandemic exacerbates existing health risks (note Neis et al. 2021). Work providing communal housing for mobile workers makes physical distancing difficult if not impossible. People of colour in the US comprise 60 per cent of warehouse/delivery workers and 74 per cent of cleaners. Ethnic minorities have had greater numbers infected and dying from COVID-19. The UK is in a similar position with black people dying of coronavirus at twice the rate as white people (Paremoer et al. 2021). However, the consequences of precarious work are greater in a country like India. Lockdown meant migrant workers lost income and had to return to their villages (with complicating factors such as financial distress, starvation, a lack of access to medical care and police brutality).

Changes in the way that work is carried out

There were a series of affirmations over whether COVID-19 had made remote work the norm (BBC 2020). This included whether workers would return to the office again. Also, what will be the effect of a 'hybrid' model on communication and connections between people? Further, will working from home create gender equality and diversity? What effect will the virtual office have if face-to-face social interactions were lost? Will vulnerable workers miss out on safety nets, and will the digital future mean that large sections of global populations are left behind?

In investigating work futures Ancillo, del Val and Gavrila (2021) undertook a documentary analysis and data search on organisational and employee experiences of remote working during COVID-19. It showed this practice has altered how organisations and employees work requiring constant reevaluation. Key transitional points are work, safety and technology.

A large Finnish study (24,299 employees) found there were significant ways that work had changed during the pandemic (Ervasti et al. 2021). It was understood that the virus had led to much work being carried out at home but the effects on well-being and workers' views of psychosocial hazards were not known. However, change can negatively affect well-being. In their study the researchers (2021) found that due to the pandemic

44 per cent of study participants had work transferred to home, while a small proportion had new tasks, and had their work team reorganised. Those moving to home-based work were mainly men and those with higher socio-economic status and lower levels of risk factors. Workers experiencing task or team reorganisation were more likely to be female with lower socio-economic status. Overall, their study found working at home led to some improved perceptions of psychosocial work factors. However new tasks and team set-ups were related to a decline in psychosocial benefits and health. They argue their results show a polarisation of work between those onsite and those at home. It also needs to be seen in the context of employees in higher echelons having the opportunity to work at home compared to those lower in the status hierarchy. This further emphasises opportunities for increased well-being and health for the more privileged.

The arrangement for remote and hybrid working would be more favoured for non-manual work after coronavirus has finished according to Vyas (2022). It will not be the case for everyone. Work practices pre-pandemic will remain after the pandemic for many workers. Much manual labour will continue with previous practices. However, the role of automation may affect this. Employers will focus on motivation and well-being. There were changes underway pre-pandemic that will continue but at a faster pace due to COVID-19; new and innovative practices will become the new normal. There will be practices modified from pre-pandemic times.

The reliance on technology for work during COVID-19

There have been major changes in human behaviour and in 'technology diffusion' due to COVID-19 (Vargo et al. 2020). A lot of activities such as learning, working and shopping moved online. This has bought about the diffusion of digital technologies for ordinary people, producing a pronounced digital divide (see Chapter 7, this volume). Donelle et al. (2023) refer to the upsurge of digital technologies during coronavirus. Vargo et al. (2020) found that a range of computerised tomography machines, video communication platforms, artificial intelligence (AI) and digital technologies were used in healthcare and other domains. Main users are teachers/students, doctors/patients, the government and the public. Health services and communication were the major users of healthcare technology: in education the main technology used was transitioning to online from face-to-face communication; and in daily use most technology was for analysing data, tracing, prediction and diagnosing COVID-19. Vargo et al. (2020) argue that the effects of new technologies which need researching include AI and the use of Zoom and related technologies. There are efforts needed to monitor access to technology and its utilisation in under-privileged areas and in developing countries. Negative effects of technology require research and monitoring, including disinformation, misinformation, privacy, cybersecurity and terrorism.

Technology is having unprecedented effects as its use increased enormously through the pandemic. Work became home based with the use of online technologies for many workers. This has meant that 'Zoom' or 'Teams' for example are used to facilitate online interaction. There has been substantial upgrading of information and communication technology (ICT) skills, and the use of metrics for monitoring, and placing new surveillance on employees. Being able to work from home dramatically reduces the support base for looking after physical and mental health and in maintaining a healthy routine. Davis, Gent and Gregory (2021) argue that the adopted style of working from home increased productivity, leading to greater lifetime incomes. They maintain the pandemic has sped up a process that would have occurred naturally.

Tens of millions around the world worked from home due to lockdowns, isolation and quarantine. This has continued since the peak of the pandemic. As an experiment it did not gain traction before COVID-19 (Lund et al. 2020). The benefits and limitations of working remotely have become clearer. Twenty per cent of workers could now work remotely, meaning three to four times the number before the pandemic.

Strict lockdowns were imposed by some governments during COVID-19 to reduce transmission of the virus and release pressure on hospital systems. People were urged to stay at home and reduce face-to-face contact with others. The WHO released a risk assessment tool for mass gatherings. It covers 'Risk Evaluation; Risk Mitigation; and Risk Communication' (Vyas and Butakhieo 2021). A total score is calculated on the risk of transmission. Employers were also encouraged to carry out a coronavirus-specific risk assessment at the workplace. They argue that one region, Hong Kong, did not undertake a strict lockdown. However, it did have measures such as limiting public assemblies as well as for schools and remote working arrangements for civil servants and encouraged the private sector to do so.

In 1973 the terms 'telecommuting' and 'telework' were first coined. This form of work has also been called flexible workplace, remote work and e-working. These terms all refer to working from home using technology. These modes are claimed to lead to increased productivity and engagement and reduced turnover, increased job satisfaction and reduced work and rest of life conflict (Vyas and Butakhieo 2021). There are some disadvantages, which include blurring the line between family and work, increased isolation and in some cases increased costs for workers (such as internet and electricity). The researchers maintain the relationships between co-workers could be harmed and young children at home could form a distraction.

While there are some positive outcomes of remote work for employees there are some negative aspects such as a heavy reliance on technologies. In a study of 1,620 people by Molino et al. (2020) the properties of a 'technostress' (stress experienced by end users of technology) scale during COVID-19 were investigated. In Italy several companies intended to keep remote work as it showed improvements in job performance, cut down travel and led to higher job satisfaction. Consequences of stress due to technology use include users reporting being under time pressure, not completing tasks on time, being an effort to be efficient much of the time and dealing with information faster. There is also the expectation that workers are fully connected and available. Molino et al. (2020) report reduced productivity and work performance (compared to other studies showing increased productivity), less job satisfaction and commitment to the organisation, lower intended ICT use and increased intentions to leave the job. These were as consequences of technostress. Further, work and life and work and family conflicts as well as job overload have been found. The results of their study supported previous studies showing that remote workers spend more time working and experience more overload and intrusion of their work into their personal life. Employees working remotely showed negative relations with work and family conflict, and stress as well as being exhausted from work.

Those working from home had to acclimatise overnight, relying on technology (Lal, Dwivedi and Haag 2021). Social interactions had been a fundamental part of work and had shaped work experience: they now had to be reconfigured to be supported by technology. The effects of this approach to technologies are yet under researched. Social interactions are a major feature of work for many employees but during COVID-19 many were confined to digital platforms for this.

Lal et al. (2021) highlighted workers' experiences and modes of collegiate social interaction in their study of 29 people working full-time from home due to the virus. They used an interpretivist framework and diary-keeping as a method of research. They focussed on the workers' social interactions using different technologies and saw these interactions as a fundamental part of their work. Using technology meant that emotional intelligence and social cues were not used. In the context of feeling negative about working from home some people in the study felt that on returning to the workplace social interactions may be seen as a distraction. Workers around the globe have been having virtual morning teas and after work zooming. It is not fully known how digital tools can alleviate isolation. Also, there are challenges in the maintenance of organisational culture when workers are communicating at a distance. A key question is, can a technology be used to preserve communication at work and socially, to maintain organisational culture (Lal et al. 2021)? Fifty-two per cent of people in their study reported they had work-based social interaction from home. However, many were quite negative about the experience. For example, one said 'I feel like the proportion of casual/personal conversations I am having with colleagues is a lot smaller when working from home (i.e., nearly all conversations are about work matters). For example, today all messages I exchanged with colleagues were about work. Without the casual conversations to break the day up, it can give the workday a more serious feel.' Only five workers said their social interaction had improved at home using technology. For example, 'I must say that I think I get more interaction with people now than when in the office… and enjoyed it today.' Whether overall they did or did not enjoy working from home, several of the workers said they missed face-to-face contact with colleagues. The range of platforms could also be a challenge. As one said, 'awareness of the use of these new social and collaboration platforms – Microsoft Teams, Skype for Business, WebEx, Zoom, Google Duo etc…can be quite overwhelming at times when people are trying to connect to you through different modes.' Overall, technology was a challenge with some suffering from technology overload and generally many people spending too much time learning and adjusting to new technology.

There are key areas in which COVID-19 is reconstituting technology's future, especially in healthcare (Queen 2021). Remote work can lead to greater productivity, 31 per cent of remote workers reported having to deal with mental health issues and 'needed a day off' while 29 per cent said they had problems managing a work and life balance during the pandemic (AKIXI 2021). Extensive use of online conferencing led to some detachment and isolation. More security is required over the longer period.

Social construction of risk with technology

The social construction of technology emerged along with the sociology of technology during the 1980s and has had a mixed impact (Basu 2023). There are several social factors that people construct in understanding risk. People behave differently in relation to the same information based on their construction of how they understand risk (Frank 2019). According to Dake (1992) culture gives socially constructed stories about nature, even though people have concerns and perceive risks. These stories or myths are internalised by people, influencing their worldviews and interpretations. Another perspective on risk is by Burns and Machado (2010) who say in democratic societies, there is public awareness and discussion of the limits of knowing and controlling technology and some risks related. Risk leads to political aspects of technology coming to the fore and scepticism of many technological developments. Writing some time ago, Nelkin (1989) argues that evaluating technological risk needs 'interpretive judgement' in the context of uncertainty. Risk communication involves social responsibility.

Klein and Kleinman (2002) refer to the agency versus structure debate when looking at the social construction of technology. Agency refers to where individual can shape the growth and development of technology. This has many proponents. The structure approach refers to the social forces which shape technological development, such as social class and inequity. Klein and Kleinman (2002) look at political economy and organisational sociology for structural factors affecting technology: these include in the design, development and transformation of the technology. They argue the social role in shaping technological development is a key factor for consideration.

Due to the coronavirus pandemic, there have been rapid advances in technology, the pace of which have left many unprepared. In terms of the social construction of technology and risk involved there are many factors contributing to difficulties in adjusting to its development. The work from home mandate meant that many had to learn innovative technologies as a way of acclimatising to the new demands of their jobs. The increased use of metrics appears to have given new powers to management and can lead to a level of alienation. Developments in automation in the time of COVID-19 have placed some jobs in jeopardy and required learning of new skills. Social factors affecting this were based in pre-existing inequities.

Pietrocola et al. (2021) refer to the work of Ulrich Beck on risk situations producing 'goods' and 'bads' in *Risk Society* (1992). They refer to COVID-19 as causing a consideration of science education's role in teaching the population regarding global risks from socio-economic development. This relates to a belief in science of coronavirus being strongly adhered to by many governments, policymakers and citizens. Yet along with other global phenomena a shared belief in science is not strong.

Ahmed et al. (2021) maintain that in the initial stages of the pandemic vaccines were not available, so physical distancing was vital, particularly at mass gatherings. It minimised human contact and overcame virus spread. It was especially important for those at high risk of infection. The co-authors presented a 'deep-learning platform' for physical distancing. They developed a detection algorithm. A tracking algorithm detects people such as those who crosses the physical distance threshold: that being a violation of minimum physical distance. A person breaching the distancing threshold is tracked. On testing, the model could distinguish which person was physically too near.

Effects of COVID-19 on work and sociopsychological health

COVID-19 has had a drastic effect on work and work environments. In healthcare mental health of workers declined. There are major factors that have affected work life, including workload, fear of becoming ill and negative effects of lockdowns contributing to 'tangible changes' in work. (Ervasti et al. 2021). Coronavirus has shown how important work is in its effects on health. Peters et al. (2022) argue that work changes have intensified due to the virus. Government organisations needed to monitor and evaluate these changes. Worker and organisation hardiness was needed to accommodate these changes into a post-COVID environment.

Post-pandemic is likely to see stress, poor self-esteem and poor mental and physical health due to unemployment. This is for young people who may have lost years in education and work because of severe economic downturns (Peterson 2021a). Some young people are at greatest risk of COVID-19 mitigation effects leading to reduced employment and educational opportunities. Governments are likely to have spent at high levels during coronavirus and have less tax resources for welfare programmes and social care. Risk is associated with economic downturns and with the extensive use of technologies can, for some, exacerbate problems.

The pandemic brought with it uncertainty: this can lead to stress and undermine performance (Saleem, Malik and Qureshi 2021). It can lead to health problems such as interpersonal conflicts damaging patterns of work and decreasing performance. Worse stress may lead to undermining workers' well-being. In their study of bank employees who had to attend work during COVID-19 the researchers (2021) found employees experiencing stress felt decreased autonomy and that they may not be performing to a required standard. Those working in risky environments also looked for pay increases, and if they were not forthcoming when working in a threatening environment, these would decrease productivity. Health hazards also lead to work absences and turnover. However, under some circumstances the stress experienced by workers in confronting new challenges may lead to increased work performance. Saleem et al. (2021) refer to a study in the US of hotel employees who found coronavirus a motivator for increased work performance.

On March 16 and 22, 2020, Switzerland followed by Germany entered full lockdown with strict measures in place until the end of April. An online survey of Swiss and German workers by Tušl et al. (2021) focussed on how COVID-19 had affected their work and personal lives. Thirty per cent reported a worsening of work and personal life (with 10% reporting that work had improved). Working from home was related to positive effects on home life, while short-term work had a poor effect on work life. Negative effects on personal life were associated with being younger, living alone, having less leisure time and having changes in caring arrangements. Positive effects on personal life were related to being in a family/partnership and having more leisure.

Nurses play important roles in preventing infection in infection control, and in isolation and containment during COVID-19. On March 1, 2020, 28,679 nurses went to Hubei Province in China engaging against the virus. One-third of deaths during the 2003 China's SARS outbreak were healthcare workers. Many in Hubei in 2020 were infected due to the virus, with 40 per cent in hospitals and 60 per cent in the community (Mo et al. 2020). The emergency in Wuhan (in the Hubei province) placed enormous pressure on nurses in an environment of high demand and few resources. This led to heightened stress and symptomatology (physical and mental) adversely affecting well-being and health. Nurses who were the 'only child' were more stressed. They feared if they died parents would be disadvantaged. This created multiple role conflicts. By strengthening nurses' social support, the effect of job strain could reduce. Nurses needed to be in touch with family and friends to gain 'spiritual support.'

Nurses and patients felt helpless due to the spread of COVID-19. The Chinese government has addressed mental health concerns (according to Mo et al. 2020). Those health workers infected with the virus while performing their duties have been recognised as having an industrial injury and have the benefit of claiming insurance; occupational injury insurance is a 'protection umbrella' for preventing and rescuing staff affected by coronavirus pneumonia. Nurse managers should assist nurses to adjust their psychological state, with leisure activities and relaxation provided.

Kim and Yang (2023) argue that during COVID-19 stress was reported by 6.3 per cent of nurses, together with anxiety (20.6%) and moderate-to-severe depression (8.5%). Other studies have shown higher figures including 29.1 per cent at risk of Post-Traumatic Stress Disorder (PTSD). The co-workers reported on an online survey of differences between COVID-19-dedicated and non-dedicated nurses. For COVID-dedicated nurses, factors influencing mental health were 'purpose and meaning,' 'perceived stigma,' 'work environment improvement' and 'absolute work intensity.' For non-dedicated nurses the only predictors of mental health were purpose and meaning and absolute work intensity. The results signified that more attention was needed on the work environment for COVID-19-dedicated nurses.

Conclusion

Economically COVID-19 has stretched the resources of most developed countries, but for nations, such as in Africa the consequences have been devastating. Activities such as tourism, so important to many countries, had just been starting to revive after three or more years. But for some nations recovery may take much longer.

The consequences in the long term of changes to work practices are becoming more evident, but it is also clear that those who endured the most negative consequences are the vulnerable and those whose work is precarious (as well as the unemployed). Owing to the influences of neoliberal policies well-defined groups usually at risk were at greater risk of death and illness and poor economic and social well-being due to coronavirus. Work at home is often for the more socioeconomically privileged and is not possible for many workers. Less advantaged workers face increased risk. However, work at home or hybrid arrangements are likely to be part of the foreseeable future.

7 The growth of digitisation, metrics and automation

This chapter investigates the growth of technology, the development of digitisation and impacts on the labour process. Three theoretical positions in relation to digitisation are discussed. Also, it will present the way in which coronavirus disease-19 (COVID-19) affected the development and spread of digitisation globally, as the speed of growth is vastly influencing many areas of life. Further, technological developments are playing a crucial role in emerging and current global issues, for example global warming/climate change. The relationship of digitisation and the pandemic is discussed, together with types of technologies and digitisation outcomes. The use of technology and digitisation has increased substantially because of COVID-19 with much work now being performed in the home as well as the need for integrated digital systems being required in healthcare.

The growth of technology and digitisation during COVID-19 has been likened to a ship in a storm. 'Against the darkness of the COVID-19 storm, a flickering light gives glimpses of the power of data and digital tools to protect and improve health and wellbeing and inspires hope of what is to come' (Horgen et al. 2020). In 2020 there was extensive digitisation, but much had remained unused in the initial stages of the pandemic. Telemedicine has become significant in healthcare and data tracking and surveillance of outbreaks has assumed a significant role for governments. Much, according to the researchers, is still needed in the search for reliable digital health technology. Data harmonisation and optimum data sharing, and analysis are required, and the adoption of 'innovative digital tools.' 'The more noble course is for orders to be given to complete the preparations, to cast off and set sail, and to join other vessels crewed by valiant healthcare workers and tireless researchers, already deeply engaged in a rescue mission for the whole of the human race' (Horgen et al. 2020).

We have moved into the age of digitisation where technology has become dominant. According to Ulrich Beck the dominant forces of science and technology are important components in risk society. Ulrich Beck described that we live in risk society (Beck 1992) within reflexive modernity (Beck, Giddens and Lash 1994; note Jong 2022). Main issues have included developing new technologies to manage the risks posed by existing technologies (Pietrocola

DOI: 10.4324/9781003449423-9

et al. 2021). Risks result from human action. Uncertainty, in Beck's view, isn't because of new knowledge and technologies, but is social and results from patterns of life and work (Burgess, Wardman and Mythen 2018). Beck argues that in late modernity society is confronted by a common issue related to the influence of a highly 'technical-scientific world.' Bertilsson (1990, 141) points out that compared to earlier times 'risks are endogenous to modern living' (meaning they are innate to or derived from) and result from technical, scientific and industrial ingenuity in taming the forces of nature.

The labour process of digital technology

Richard Baldwin's (2019a, b) work on digitalisation, automation and 'globotics' pre-coronavirus established some important aspects of the accelerated growth of technology. There has been an exponential growth in technology. Baldwin addresses issues of control in the workplace which have implications for the labour process particularly for those workers involved with information and communication technology (ICT). Whereas a common conception might be that technology can bring a loss of control for workers, many employed in ICT have increased their control over their jobs due to growth in technical skill and expertise. They may know more than their bosses. This increase in control shows quite a different trend to assumptions that technology will disempower workers.

Due to COVID-19 and its effects through lockdowns workers, government and companies have sped up the process of implementing the technology. Forslid and Baldwin (2020) maintain the focus is usually on developed nations, but they may transform economic development. 'Globotics' (that is robotics and globalisation) can 'disable' the Chinese style based on manufacturing and 'enable' the services development model that India is engaged with.

According to Briken et al. (2017) digitisation in the workplace has supervisors monitoring not only customers, but employees. Prospective employees need to be technologically competent. Prior to COVID-19 digitised workplaces would bring about changes in skills, employment patterns, control and autonomy. Metrics are more ways of recording outputs and productivity of workers. They are also used as a mechanism of surveillance of workers. Their increased use can lead to a decrease in power and control of workers. Jarvis (2021) discusses the rise of metrics in academic labour and the effects it has had on the labour process. They have reduced outcomes of much academic labour to quantitative categories, when a more qualitative-based understanding is required.

Klur and Nies (2023) base their analysis of digitation on Marx's conception of the 'role of technology as a means of domination,' and that machinery in industry deskills labour. People are subjected to the speed of the machines, not freeing the worker but making work uninteresting (Marx 2010). Employees do not have power to dispose of the means of production. Klur and

Nies (2023) wanted to use a Marxist framework for analysing digital technology. However, 'digital self-perpetuation doesn't follow the machine cycle' or Fordist assembly line logic. They are based on increasing productivity. 'Rather, digital self-perpetuation here follows a logic of the market economy – because digital technology in our cases essentially serves to link production to the market and, thereby, responds to the new demands of post-Fordist capitalism' (Klur and Nies 2023, 27).

Lopez et al. (2022) look at labour process in value chain restructuring. In the face of digital competition, fast-fashion retailers 'digital value chain' managements are attempting to expand and secure market share and power of value chains. Fast-fashion retailers are looking to bring in digital supply chain management systems. Rationalisation and standardisation, deskilling and new digital types of labour control are linked to management of digital practices in retailers' digital supply chains. Gender, power relations and employees' position are factors affecting working conditions. Lopez et al. (2022) refer to digital capitalism as the way of digitally integrating and controlling the labour process.

Theoretical perspectives for digitisation

Critical public health identifies digital technologies used for control and care in surveilling COVID-19. Public health attempts to deal with population health (Lupton 2022a). It looks at socio-political issues related to public health, including digital technologies in health. In critical public health, being responsible for one's own health is important, given the stigmatisation of being ill for poor and vulnerable groups over centuries. This is the context of infection disease control.

Lupton (2020) uses three social theory perspectives on the role of digital technologies on the social, political and cultural aspects of coronavirus. Firstly, based on Marx the political economy approach looked at social class and social structure and related inequalities. It focusses on 'disparities in benefits' of digital technologies. These are due to class, age, gender, location disability and race. During COVID-19 the political economy perspective identifies that not all people can engage with digital technologies (including apps and websites for preventative measures). Neoliberalism has protected the privileged from coronavirus. Lupton refers to 'disaster capitalism' which includes digital surveillance technologies which may result in the apportioning of blame to those seen as not being responsible citizens, even if this is due to being in poverty.

A Foucauldian perspective emphasises the productive nature of power, bringing practices and knowledge into action. 'Biopolitics and biopower refer to the complex power relations involved when state agencies such as government health departments, non-government and commercial enterprises and lay people and healthcare professionals work together to manage the health and bodies of populations' (Lupton 2020). Foucault's perspectives have looked at how groups (body politic) and individuals have been governed by COVID-19. This includes being disciplined and managed during the crisis. Apps, drones and software have been used to model disease spread and people's behaviour and health: this represents 'radical biopolitics.' Some digital technologies used by governments restricted the freedoms of people, such as apps restricting movement from the home. However, this was in the context of trying to control the virus, to ensure health and economic well-being for society. These measures were more than attempts at political control.

The third theoretical approach described by Lupton is more than human theory, or 'new managerialism.' It refers to where collectives are formed between humans and nonhumans (e.g. plant, animals, landscapes, water, food). In COVID-19 there have been pandemic assemblages which change constantly. The virus resulted from animals in a wet market infecting humans in China. Some of the spread of coronavirus occurred when humans touched surfaces (nonhuman element). 'Together, these human and nonhuman agents generated affective forces and agencies that enhanced or diminished humans' capacities for action' (Lupton 2020). Feelings of helplessness and low control represent ways people interacted with apps, digital messaging, telemedicine and other forms of digital health technologies during the virus. This includes social media, telemedicine and video streaming while working from home, and ways of maintaining contact with others. This more than human perspective shows the importance of non-digitised responses (e.g. use of masks, presence of warning signs) to the use of digital technologies during coronavirus, in understanding the impact of digital responses. Further there needs to be sociological research on the sociopsychological impacts of digital technologies during their roll-out for COVID-19. Also, research is needed on which mediums were most helpful, and their impact on the healthcare system.

COVID-19 and digitisation

Abidi, El Herradi and Sakha (2022) maintain that digitisation is a way of businesses minimising losses due to coronavirus. Metrics are being used as ways of recording outputs and productivity of workers: their increased use can lead to a decrease in power and control of workers. In Australia digitisation is the way forward for businesses to survive and grow. The use of technology and digitisation has increased enormously because of COVID-19 with much work being performed in the home and integrated digital systems being required in healthcare.

Horgen et al. (2020) maintain that sharing information has been argued for repeatedly, and information transparency and acting collectively were essential in dealing with the pandemic. Technology in fighting the virus is still not used to its potential, however, even though it plays a key role in mitigating against the virus. Rapid data sharing is important. There is a need for government, industry and academia to collaborate and this will give a better understanding of what digital data can bring.

OECD (2021b) outlines the impact of COVID-19 on technology, science and innovation, in research organisations, firms, universities and science and technology organisations. The speed of innovation due to coronavirus has had a major impact. The uptake of digital tools and associated technology has accelerated as has the inclusiveness of innovation systems. COVID-19 could lead to experimenting with new tools, policies and modes of governance. The OECD reported that coronavirus threatened to cause damage over the long term to action on other global emergencies such as global warming/climate change and in addressing sustainable futures.

In a review of digital technologies employed during COVID-19, Budd et al. (2020) focussed on their uses in public health, including surveillance of populations, identification of cases, evaluation of interventions and contact tracing. Some of the barriers to their implementation include ethical, legal and privacy, as well as organisational issues. They (2020) maintain the future of public health is increasingly digital, as is being prepared for future pandemics and other global issues. As a way of contrast public health measures such as isolation and restricting human movement were also used in the 14th-century European plague. We live in a digital era. By 2019 65 per cent of mobile devices were smartphones with major growth in Sub-Saharan Africa region. Some 3.8 billion globally used social media. In 2023 there were 5.19 billion or 64.5 per cent of the world's population using the Internet, and 5.56 billion or 69.8 per cent as unique mobile phone subscribers (Digital Around the World 2023).

Contact tracing has been successful in South Korea, China and Taiwan, except for claims of privacy and human rights violations. There are digital contact tracing apps developed around the world to help in crisis management. The digital app Smittestopp was developed in Norway for infection tracking, but despite the government performing well in crisis management, the measures for contact tracing had minor impact (Lund-Tønnesen and Christensen 2023). Version 1 of the app was declared illegal in June/July 2020 by the Norwegian Data Protection Authority based on claims of excessive intrusion into privacy. There was a second version of the app introduced in December 2020. Despite complying with strict privacy regulations, the public made little use of it. These apps represent technologies that provide governance legitimacy. Due to a low population density and high trust in government the researchers (2023) question the need to use such technology. The app was not very helpful with the crisis in Norway. The 'initial input and throughput legitimacy' is crucial if government's policy is to keep 'output legitimacy' and provide effective governance in a crisis.

In advanced economies, COVID-19 accelerated digitalisation, that is with workers using a computer with internet access (Jaumotte et al. 2023). The largest growth was in southern and eastern Europe, and in food and accommodation, and small companies. This growth was in regions/sectors with low technology. The researchers (2023) point out that digitalisation helped with employment and productivity during coronavirus. At the peak of the virus high level digitised organisations had less hours of work lost and less loss of productivity. More digitised sectors increased productivity by 25 per cent and cut lost hours by more than 30 per cent. In 2021 these outcomes rebounded more strongly in low rather than highly digitised sectors. Employees in more digitised firms were less likely to lose their jobs. Jaumotte et al. (2023) maintain, however, there is no evidence of a structural change in the labour market favouring digitised jobs. A major change due to coronavirus was the shift to working from home. Digitisation softened the effects of shocks from the virus as well as sustaining productivity and improving workers' home and work balance.

Pirosca et al. (2021) discuss the impact of 'digital efficiency' on the labour market. Technological developments constantly have an impact. The researchers looked at the effects of digital skill levels on employees' pay in the EU. They found that pay is highly correlated with digital expertise and internet use. They conclude that digital skill enhancement can provide a more flexible labour market.

Charles, Xia and Coutts (2022) reported on digitisation and labour markets for the International Labour Organisation (ILO). COVID-19 encouraged digital transformation. Developed countries are heading for 'fast-evolving, data-driven digital economies.' This is reshaping work and the functioning of labour markets. Most countries in the OECD have digitisation strategies. Malaysia, Nigeria, Egypt and China also have digitalisation as a development strategy. It applies to many jobs. They include the 'gig' market, and on-demand logistics services, high skilled workers in remote software development and 'influencers' earning an income through social media and livestreaming. Digital workers are mainly male and young and represent an unbalanced organisation of labour. Digitisation has altered the structure of the labour market (Charles et al. 2022).

Misinformation and risk

WHO (2021b) maintains coronavirus has seen misinformation spread on digital platforms such as social media thereby making it a global public health threat. Technology and social media create an 'infodemic,' undermining the response to the virus affecting control measures. Young people are most active online and therefore are central to this, even though they are at less risk of the virus. In a survey of more than 20,000 Gen Ys and Millennials from 24 countries in early 2021 it was found that just less than half wanted to share scientific content on digital platforms (WHO 2021b). About one-third ignored 'fake news,' about 90 per cent worried about infection from coronavirus, and half were concerned about family members being infected.

Increases in being dependent on digital technologies raise questions on well-being (Kitkowska, Alaqra and Wästlund 2023). This includes when the technologies pose a threat and when are they most appreciated. Some companies modify current technologies or develop new ones if they don't satisfy end users or may pose a risk to their well-being. Kitkowska et al. (2023) studied 578 digital technology users globally. They found that many digital technologies were appreciated (such as for work and shopping). However, there were some concerns for adverse physical and mental health effects. Respondents saw the technologies emotionally as an integral part of their lives. There is a need for designers to be aware of barriers and enablers to accepting their technologies. However, it might not be able to overcome the problems related to digital well-being. Managements in work and school contexts need to look for a better distribution of activities in relation to physical and digital worlds. This could include blending online with off-screen and offline activities.

Due to technology, social support comes from a broad network. These networks have dramatically increased since the start of COVID-19 (Long et al. 2022). However, it is not clear if online networks substitute for person to person contact during physical distancing. The co-workers cite research showing that increased face to face and phone/video contact during 2020 reduced depression. They also argue that social support inequalities exist with many people having fewer opportunities for access: this was heightened by coronavirus.

Types of technologies

Lupton (2020) argues that the use of telemedicine grew dramatically when physical distancing and isolation meant limitations to visiting health providers during COVID-19. 'Digital technologies have also played an important role in population monitoring, containment and control measures' (Lupton 2020). Smartphones and 'social media' apps have been used for surveilling symptoms, for contact tracing or self-isolation and quarantine. She describes how drones have disinfected public areas and warn of isolation rule breaking (Lupton 2022b).

Digitalisation may be the greatest corporate response to coronavirus (Schaupp 2022). There has been an increase in software investment for digitising, while robotic investment remains stagnant during the COVID-19 crisis. This represents a rise of 'algorithmic management' for profitability and a substitute for automation. He refers to 'algorithmic management (as that) which encompasses the digital direction, evaluation and optimisation of labour processes' (Schaupp 2022).

WHO has encouraged governments around the globe to provide surveillance of people infected with COVID-19 to help control the spread of the virus. Technologies including robots, drones, Bluetooth and Global Positioning System (GPS) have a role to play in surveilling and controlling virus effects (Saher and Anjum 2021). Wearable devices using GPS and Bluetooth can monitor health and stress levels while isolating. Telemedicine is an effective mechanism to ensure safety against infection and has been used in medical encounters at a distance, ensuring the safety of health staff and patients.

Technologies used during COVID-19 range from masks to robots. Robot use ranged from sterilisation to delivering food to the needy. Digital technology provided practitioner groups with sharing information. Artificial intelligence (AI) has also been used in producing drugs and analyses of CT scans. One major drawback however with some technology such as AI has been the erosion of privacy and the surveillance of populations.

Outcomes of digitisation

Osler and Zahavi (2022) researched how digital communication and sociality affect our experience of others, and particularly how our experience of each other changes in digital space. Encounters in digital space represent their own type of sociality because the medium requires a phenomenological analysis of its own. The researchers (2022) argue that some senses such as touch are missing from digital encounters. Loss of tactile senses is more important for some than others. During online interactions friends or colleagues are out of reach, and it does not represent being together, particularly in strong emotional interactions. In addition, Zooms mostly show people from the shoulders up, and it may be that other body language gestures are telling a fuller story. Despite advances in technology people are physically separate. Relying more on technology to increase social encounters during coronavirus changed the structure of social experience, especially in relation to sociality, which is different to social encounters offline. Osler and Zahavi (2022) however argue, it is not the case that online sociality is only valued when it can mirror offline sociality.

Manual contact tracing is difficult when a lot of infected people are involved. Early in COVID-19 the development of several digital contact tracing tools aided the task with more options developed during the pandemic (Sideri and Prainsack 2023). Bluetooth Low Energy was the 'technical architecture' used mostly. The apps were downloadable, and this was voluntary, although many people did not do this. There were questions of privacy with the app that conflicted with public health requirements. However, the apps were deployed as a soft method to get people acting collectively. Their use has implications for future pandemics.

Digital technologies may help guard against negative outcomes of COVID-19 by reducing isolation and loneliness and providing social support. Few studies have looked at positive outcomes of these technologies during the virus. Canale et al. (2022) focussed on how positive outcomes may occur despite adversities. Italy was one of the worst affected counties with COVID-19. The co-workers looked at explaining social and personal wellbeing and advantages of using digital technologies from an online sample of 1,412 adults in 2020. They investigated the impact of restrictions due to coronavirus and found that using emotions online was associated with post-traumatic growth, good mental health and positive social behaviours. Those having greater social support online also had better mental health and social behaviours.

Marston et al. (2020) use the stress process model (see Peterson 2018) to argue that stress on economic and social well-being has occurred because of coronavirus. This includes immense disruptions to social relations. Digital technologies can be an alternative to life in lockdown to maintain social and economic activities. There is an extensive literature on increasing digital technologies including virtual conferencing and social networking sites. This shows there were different approaches to creating and enhancing social activities and connections during COVID-19. It represents a large growth area for research in the social sciences and sociology, computer science and gerontechnology.

In a Pew Research survey in the US reported by McClain et al. (2021) 90 per cent of adults said in April 2021 that the internet was important personally during their experience of the pandemic, while 58 per cent said it was essential. This was at a time when the government was starting to loosen some of the COVID-19 restrictions and when vaccinations were introduced. It was rated more important based on having more formal education, by those under 30 years and those 65 years and older. Most had spoken with others using video calls. Just less than half felt they used digital tools in new or diverse ways. Nearly 30 per cent sought upgrades to their digital services during the pandemic. About two-thirds of people surveyed felt that digital mediums did not replace face-to-face communications. 'Zoom fatigue' for many was a problem, and one-third of adults surveyed said they tried reducing time spent on their internet and smartphone. Despite the benefits of technology about 25 per cent felt less close to family than prior to coronavirus, and 38 per cent felt less connected to quite close friends, and more than half to casual acquaintances.

COVID-19 has meant people have a sense of affiliation through digital technologies and social networks. Panday et al. (2021) used qualitative methods to investigate experiences and attitudes of patients with coronavirus and their carers towards the virus. Experiences such as fear of spreading disease to others and the need for counselling were evident. Family played an important positive role. Stigmatised attitudes of neighbours were a particular problem, however. Altruistic people played a role in promoting social harmony through some tangible supports. They found digital technology played a positive role as it helped maintain social connections. Modern technology may be the only way that people can deal with isolation and fragmented social relations bought about by the pandemic.

During COVID-19 increased reliance on technology for staying connected and learning and for many, everyday functions steadily increased. Goldschmidt (2020) showed how important technology was to children's well-being when isolation and distancing became essential. The US Centre for Disease Control and Prevention had recommended supervised telephone calls and videoconference chats for children with their friends.

In virtual teaching environments universities have achieved a level of success using appropriate platforms. As a result of the virus some students had worries and fears leading to discrimination and loss. Globally, this has left these institutions in a predicament (Al-Maroof et al. 2020). Fears for students were related to the use and effectiveness of technology. This included loss of social relationships, to family lockdown and of failing at education in the context of COVID-19. After the pandemic peak it meant international students could travel to resume studies, and the Chinese government said they would no longer recognise studies gained from remote learning.

In Australia digitisation has been seen as the way forward for businesses to survive and grow. The use of technology and digitisation has increased enormously because of COVID-19 with much work now being performed in the home. There is also a need for integrated digital systems in healthcare.

Digitisation: Preparing for the future

Cyber technology (information and communication technology) has had a huge growth and at national and global levels cyber security has become particularly important (Klein and Hossein 2020). Protecting and regulating cyberspace especially from malicious use is juxtaposed with its fair use. Control and ownership of information and threats of hacking are serious issues. Government is the major proponent, but Klein and Hossein (2020) identified the impact on individuals of cyber security as a major issue. In the light of rapid advances of digitisation and the threat of climate change, the implications and security issues for individuals who live and work in the Arctic region are major. It is a region most susceptible to extremes of climate change where cyber security and the safety of information are vital.

The development of cyber security and digitisation have increased more rapidly due to COVID-19. They would have increased 'naturally' but coronavirus has hastened it. Hacking in 2023 has become a major international issue. There are some state-based hackers compromising the security and safety of many national and international systems. The future may hold many things, including pandemics such as COVID-19 and globally working together to contain climate change. Future events require advances of digitisation to deal with the enormity of information. As we have seen with coronavirus the cooperative linking of nation states, continents and the international bodies to bring about political, economic and social inputs to solutions is essential. This includes dealing with hacking.

For the future, moving to net zero in climate change needs major social, industrial and government supports requiring technological innovations. 'Digital technologies offer the potential to deliver sustained solutions to many of the seemingly intractable societal challenges relating to climate change …. (this includes having a significant role) in improving resilience to global warming related, natural hazards, reducing emissions and enhancing the ability for humans to take the necessary steps to realize net zero'

(Dwivedi et al. 2022). However, there are not all positives from developments in digitalisation. Some of the negative factors associated with providing solutions are resource usage, waste products and CO_2 emissions. Disposal of electronic waste is also an environmental problem.

Conclusion

Developments in technology and specifically in digitisation have had mixed effects on labour and the workforce whilst reducing the control of many workers. It has also been associated with increases in control for some, especially in the ICT field. COVID-19 bought with it substantial development in digitisation (and metrics), some of which would have occurred naturally but over a longer time. Increases in digitisation are part of the future and can have both positive and negative effects.

For some of the workforce working from home, or hybrid arrangements may be the way of the future. For these workers there is a premium placed on IT skills and the need to substitute face-to-face interactions with online communication. It remains to be seen the extent of stress and sociopsychological issues that emerge with the use of digital alternative to face-to-face interaction, and research so far reported confirms these will be issues to deal with.

8 Implications for the world of the management of COVID-19

There has been extensive action by nations and international bodies in combatting coronavirus. Many of these actions and mandates have had worldwide affects – these are discussed in this chapter. There have been economic measures which have included support packages in many countries as a brief return to a welfare state. Countries with emerging markets had the poorest economic effect and mortality because of coronavirus. Further, the implications of inter-government cooperation are presented, when neoliberal policy and practices have been inadequate to deal with the pandemic. Government interventions have involved some mandates. These include lockdowns, curfews, school closures, quarantining, mask wearing, mandatory mask wearing and vaccination. Technology including digitisation is discussed in this chapter, as are the effects of the virus on people's lives.

Emerging from the pandemic

World Health Organization (WHO) (2020b) maintains there needs to be recognition to 'build back better' from coronavirus, as noted by the United Nations (UN). Experience and expertise are needed to support people in achieving Sustainable Development Goals for health and food sectors. Rural poverty needs addressing in terms of more jobs, extended social protection, pathways of migration and formalising the informal economy. Environment needs rethinking with climate change as an urgent priority. This will help protect the livelihoods, health and food security and nutrition of all 'making our 'new normal .... a better one' (WHO 2020b).

Global greenhouse emissions fell by 17 per cent during the first year of coronavirus disease-19 (COVID-19) and by 26 per cent in some regions. There was cleaner air and the crime rate fell. There was also greater flexibility in how work was carried out and in green energy programmes (Gray 2020). The future after the virus could be in more sustainable economies and societies. There could be financial packages for companies to develop outputs to make better use of digitisation. Also, there could be reforms to green energy programmes and to digital technology. The three major changes to occur

DOI: 10.4324/9781003449423-10

because of the virus are developments in climate change, digital technology and health services.

Anderson, Rainie and Vogels (2021) argue that from the pandemic up to 2025 there will be more 'authoritarianism, inequality and misinformation.' These may be an extension of leadership in China, Russia and Donald Trump in the US and in the growth of populist parties in some countries.

Business will see growth from a huge wave of spending on physical assets by 2027. Women's unfair position is telling in healthcare where their performance and opportunity is better than in other sectors (McKinsey 2022a). Further there has been a learning loss for students worldwide due to COVID-19. There are also the lingering effects of the damage caused to the airline industry and massive changes to the labour market (McKinsey 2022b).

Financial incentives: Increasing the welfare state

Australia's social and economic responses to the COVID-19 pandemic focussed on some vulnerable groups. It was one of the most successful countries in dealing with the virus. Coronavirus had aggravated social inequality which may be more evident after recovery, although debate on means of dealing with that is polarising (O'Sullivan, Rahamathulla and Pawar 2020). Further debate should be careful not to exacerbate inequities that already exist.

COVID-19 posed serious threats to livelihoods. With growing unemployment and income risk, most OECD countries implemented programmes and policies to cushion rising social risks and preserve people's livelihoods (Noh, Han and Choi 2022). However, some governments spent only 1 per cent of GDP in 2020, and others over 10 per cent. All 31 OECD countries in the study increased social spending during the pandemic. The US (14.40%) spent most, then Japan (13.79%), followed by Canada (12.25%), while the UK spent 10.92 per cent of GDP. However, Nordic countries, having 'well-developed welfare states,' had comparatively low additional 'social spending' – Denmark (1.74%) as well as Finland (2.18%). France (6.92%) and Germany (9.83%) had higher than average 'additional social spending' while there was low spending by Southern and Eastern European nations. South Korea spent only 3 per cent of GDP. Liberal welfare countries spent significantly more and social democratic welfare states spent less. Countries such as the US, Canada, UK and Australia spent more. Much expenditure reflects the amount of spending in the economy. As Nordic states invest strongly in welfare their COVID-19 supplement was more modest. This compared to some countries offering less general economic protection, and so their social/welfare spending was greater. Also, there was higher government spending in countries with larger debt.

In early COVID-19 there was closing borders, workplaces and schools, lockdowns and the practices of 'self-isolation' and 'physical distancing.' There were several universal public health directives. De Groot and Lemanski

(2021) use South Africa as an example to show that being able to change one's life in relation to the coronavirus is a privilege. It is not possible to transform one's life in urban poverty when there is overcrowding. There are limitations with the virus in terms of inequity to access infrastructure: this will extend beyond the pandemic. Global public health measures have not sufficiently recognised inequities.

There are underlying economic and social factors in the pandemic due to the neoliberal order and the crisis resulting. This occurred as the post-war welfare state was dismantled. COVID-19 showed up the inadequacy of 'market-based solutions.' Further, there could be a return to the welfare state (at least to some degree), rather than retaining a free market approach. The pandemic has shown that rather than just being a health issue it has a social, political, economic and geographic form. Neoliberalism has failed to prepare for the pandemic, contain the virus, has led to privatising health and has exacerbated inequities. It has focussed on individual responsibilities, failed to secure jobs, and provided low levels of protection (Budzi 2022). Corona-virus required decisive action. The whims of market mechanisms have been exposed. Beyond coronavirus, the researcher proposes there needs to be a move 'towards the welfare state' with the state having a key role in economic and social aspects.

Inter-government cooperation

OECD (2020b) reports there have been heterogeneous effects of the COVID-19 crisis affecting policy and crisis management responses. These have had financial, health and economic consequences. National and subnational government organisations must deal with 'territorial effects' of corona-virus. There have also been positive outcomes from 'multi-level governance.'

Population health is affected more in some areas than others. Deprived areas are more affected. In the US late in 2020 rural counties had higher death rates. According to OECD (2020b) this requires a territorial approach by policymakers. It needs a strong inter-governmental coordinated action. There was massive fiscal support for households, businesses and the vulnerable. There were large investment recovery initiatives by some governments. The pandemic led to activating multi-level governance and public investment to build resistance and promote inter-regional and inter-municipal collaboration as well as cooperation across borders. In addition, it limited the deteriorating circumstances of vulnerable groups. COVID-19 led to shared data and evidence. It also involved reviewing subnational spending and financing to restore financial stability. In terms of developing resilience, it bought social and climate objectives into planning at all government levels: this was to ensure recovery from coronavirus and to allocate funding for public investment at all government levels.

Researchers have focussed on coronavirus effects on financial markets and the global economy. Unemployment, reduced services and transport disruptions had most governments underestimating the effects of virus risks. Pak et al. (2020) called for cooperative international action: '(w)ith globalisation, urbanization, and environmental change, infectious disease outbreaks and epidemics have become global threats requiring a collective response.' North American and European countries have real-time surveillance and health resources to combat the spread of infectious diseases. Public health capacity in countries with elevated risk needed national and international support to build and finance platforms to combat the spread of disease. This includes gaining resources to speed up research and development.

Coronavirus changed relationships between the state, society and the market in G-7 countries (Canada, France, Germany, Italy, Japan, UK, US and EU) and further afield. Shutdown caused economies to collapse with the 'state and civil society' protecting people from harmful effects of the virus. This led to a change in public perception of the governing bases for wellness in society. During coronavirus the economic response dropped, while environmentally there were reduced CO_2 emissions, but greater waste from disposable gloves and clothing (De Miranda and Snower 2021).

Jones, Palumbo and Brown (2021) report that the pandemic left businesses and economies reviewing the costs. After a year there was no way of knowing when the coronavirus would end, and what the world would look like. During the virus millions of workers were recipients of 'government-based job retention schemes.' There was a standstill in hospitality and tourism. In Australia job vacancies returned to pre-pandemic levels, but not so for Spain, France and the UK. In 2020 China was the only major economy to grow, and they and India were behind global growth in 2021. One area that has developed out of lockdown is online shopping.

There was an enormous international scientific response in dealing with coronavirus to 'understand viral genetics, immunopathogenesis, and therapeutic strategies' (Hiscott et al. 2020). Private and public funders have supported multidisciplinary projects about addressing the 'detection, treatment and prevention' of the virus. The national level is not sufficient to deal with pandemics. Networks worldwide have connected physical and social/behavioural scientists, and those in bioinformatics and engineering. Companies manufacturing perfume during the coronavirus were producing disinfectants and hand sanitisers. Others started to make face masks, and some switched to making ventilators. These contributions to fighting the virus represented a new level of national and international cooperation and collaboration. These included non-virology scientists allowing the use of their laboratories as diagnostic testing centres for the virus. 'This pandemic has also brought to light the importance of open science, data-sharing and new means of communication among members of the scientific community' (Hiscott et al. 2020). Public datasets are now available, with the need for accuracy being high, requiring greater scrutiny. Scientists welcomed this data sharing and newer forms of communication.

Effects of government mandates

There were several mandates enacted by governments across the globe. These include lockdowns, in some cases curfews, physical distancing, mask-wearing, self-isolation and vaccination.

Since early in the pandemic some researchers hoped for major changes in post-COVID-19 times. These included greater attention to climate change and the potential of new political and social orders. After a year of major disruptions and social changes, isolation, impacts of infections, restrictions to travel and moving into virtual space there were questions of how, in future, this will affect science. There were issues also about how concerns such as the Black Lives Matter movement and the postcolonial critique raise question about researchers' power relations and dominant concepts in academia (Dittmer and Lorenz 2022).

Detrimental effects of lockdowns have affected many including elite athletes. A survey of 76 world class athletes was based on stress experienced and dietary habit changes reported while they were in lockdown and in 'bubble training camps' (Washif et al. 2021). Only minor changes in stress were reported (more in bubble camps than lockdown). Older athletes, males, married, those with less experience, para-athletes and specific ethnic groups were most affected by lockdown (e.g. through increased stress). However, the researchers (2021) report the opposite effects for bubble camps. Sociodemographics, better training routines, level of well-being and diet explained more than one quarter of reduced stress on a bubble camp. These latter factors have implications for reduced stress. In lockdown, bubble camps provided some benefits.

Lockdown and similar control measures were successful in containing the spread of the virus. For example, Yuan et al. (2020) studied preventative measures to combat COVID-19 in mainland China. From January 23, 2020, there was no travel in or out of Wuhan. Using a regression model, they estimated by delaying control measures by three days the number of cases outside of Wuhan would have increased the confirmed cases by 34.6 per cent. Bringing in controls by three days would lead to 30.8 per cent less infections, or 48.6 per cent with the use of extremely strict measures. The researchers found that measures used in Wuhan as well as country-wide travel restrictions and self-isolation had the effect of reducing the spread of coronavirus in China.

The effect of the virus and delayed access to emergency departments influenced outcomes of emergency surgery. Ciarleglio et al. (2021) looked at pre-pandemic figures compared to the Italian national lockdown in March–May 2020. They found that during COVID-19 there was 'poorer prognoses,' and morbidity rates were higher. Due to the fear of infection only the most severe cases came to the emergency department in time. Control measures had some quite negative consequences. A survey of Austrians found that the use of lockdowns for four weeks had some detrimental effects on psychological health, including coping strategies. Budimir, Probst and Pieh (2021) found that so-cial support, positive thinking and using active coping led to a higher psy-chological quality of life. Those with higher levels of coping with COVID-19 had the best mental health in lockdown. Positive thinking, followed by social support, was best for mental health. Positive coping skills were related to lower depression and distress during the pandemic.

Essential labour

A major coronavirus issue in Europe was could there be a guarantee on the supply of workers, considered as key to social and economic function, or of essential labour? This included mobile workers. They were regarded as 'secondary' components of the labour market, employed precariously and were mainly migrants. Could the supply of these workers be sustained, while public health had measures such as border closures and lockdowns (Berntsen and Marino 2023)? European countries resorted to using 'emergency' inter-ventions. With air traffic halted Austria flew in migrant workers anyway. Regardless of lockdowns, between Germany and Rumania an air bridge was set up to fly in Rumanian workers. In the UK there were emergency proce-dures established for mobile EU workers. Despite considerable anti-migrant sentiment these practices during COVID-19 show how important migrant labour is. The pandemic highlights the role of the states in facilitating mi-grant workers across national borders to meet the needs of employers. Yet, during coronavirus, the states did little to protect these workers' rights. The states had relaxed restrictions for these workers, allowed 'fly-ins,' gave them residency status during the virus emergency, quickly lifted work restrictions and hastened naturalisation applications. However, little has been done to address the exploitation of migrant labour. Coronavirus exposed the states' needs for this type of labour. New state policies need to address opportunistic practices by employers to recruit these workers. This is at a time when less than standard working conditions and monitoring fair employment policies and exploitation remained.

Vaccination

Weinberger (2021) reports on the use of vaccinations for older people to maintain healthy ageing, to avoid healthcare and meet social and economic challenges. Several vaccines are recommended in many countries for older people. In the SARS-CoV-2 pandemic older people were some of the first targeted for vaccination due to the risk of severe illness. Older adults, those with underlying co-morbidities and those who are obese, have higher risk of severe illness and death from the virus. In 2021 there were long-lasting effects of the virus. The vaccines needed to be efficient to control the pandemic. Most vaccination programmes at a national level target older adults. Several vaccines have been licensed across a number of countries with clinical trials ongoing. In future years, Weinberger (2021) argues SARS-CoV-2 vaccines may be part of 'national vaccination schedules' for the entire population or alternatively for at risk groups. In 2021 the first studies were instigated for co-administering of SARS-CoV-2 vaccines with influenza, for example, or pneumococcal vaccines and developing a combination of vaccines.

'Trust and misinformation' helped shape COVID-19 and vaccine perceptions in ethnic minority groups in Scotland. Adekola et al. (2022) reported on building trust and vaccine engagement and confidence. To understand these issues there must be a focus on underlying misinformation and trust. Ethnic minority groups have proportionately high rates of coronavirus infections and deaths. Conflicting information gained from scientific and non-scientific sources, the extent of information and its sources, conspiracy theories and policy and risk inconsistencies all contributed to misinformation about COVID-19. Sources aiding perception of risk and safety included science, pharmaceutical companies and government, as well as the uptake of vaccine. Different mediums and languages are needed to convey these messages. This problem will not disappear post-pandemic. It needs following through to mitigate the effects of inequity and disadvantage for groups like the ethnic minorities. Future pandemic responses will also require measured responses, based on what we have learned through this pandemic.

The COVID-19 pandemic has shown it is important to understand and translate vaccine availability to improvements in health policy (Attwell 2023). The researcher plans to use coronavirus mandates and develop policy while collaborating with decision-makers for future vaccine preparation. They will use multiple methodologies to track effects of vaccine mandates into the future.

Economic effects

Alon et al. (2023) investigated the macroeconomic effects of coronavirus globally through income distribution. They compared low-income countries (such as Bangladesh, Ethiopia, Somalia), emerging markets (e.g. India, Brazil, China) and countries with advanced economies (such as Canada, France, Australia), as classified by the International Monetary Fund (IMF). Emerging markets had the poorest macroeconomic effect and public health outcomes. Their Gross Domestic Product (GDP) reduced by 6.7 per cent over 2019–20 while advanced economies reduced by 2.4 per cent with a 3.6-per cent reduction in low-income countries. Mortality patterns were similar with Alon et al. (2023) reporting excess mortality 75 per cent higher in emerging economies contrasted with advanced economies. There also appears to be a lower mortality rate in countries with a low income. Emerging markets had high levels of employment in jobs needing social interaction. In addition, people in households that were economically vulnerable kept working rather than staying in the safety of their home. Younger people in low-income countries were less likely to succumb to the virus. Also, much work is in agriculture and that has fewer social interactions.

Age effects

Ninety-five per cent of those in the US who died from coronavirus were aged 50 years or older. Eighty per cent were aged 65 years or older. This loss will remain long after COVID-19 has gone according to Sorrell (2021). With lockdowns and having visitors restricted isolation with declining health could lead to a lonely death. There are ageist stereotypes with older people often viewed as a burden. Older people who died from the virus in nursing homes had substantial changes in routines through lockdowns with family visits, eating together, and engaging in group activities halted. Lockdowns and restrictions on visitors meant a 'frightening isolation' which often led to poorer health or death.

There have been several inequalities leading to hardship during the pandemic. Race is just one. Pearman et al. (2022) reported on a study of stress, anxiety and depression during COVID-19 from October to November 2020 in the US. They found that the experience of stress depended on age and race. Older rather than younger Whites experienced more stress, while more Black Americans of any age experienced it compared to Whites. Older Whites reported more anxiety in relation to COVID-19, while systemic racism has a stronger effect than age for Black adults. The patterns of vulnerabilities and inequality that emerged into the pandemic are not likely to recede post-COVID-19.

Increased use of technology and digitisation

With improved technology due to the pandemic substantial improvements may occur in workplaces, social activities and with healthcare. However, by 2023 globally there have been shortages in staff for healthcare and in many cases shortages of medical supplies. In Australia for example wait times for Emergency Medicine, and for General Practitioners (GPs), have ballooned out as have availability for some pharmaceuticals due to problems with supply lines. In the short term there will be deeper relationships forged with technology due to reliance on it during COVID-19. Work, commerce, education, healthcare and social life will engage more with digitisation (Anderson, Rainie and Vogels 2021). However, there will be more inequity due to technological development. The impact and power of large firms will increase especially through developments in artificial intelligence (AI). Further social divisions will bring more misinformation.

During COVID-19 eating in restaurants suffered but several food home delivery organisations fared very well. Some companies provided remote services of their core businesses. Also, based on stay-at-home during the virus customers have engaged in digital interactions with firms (Joby and Thakur 2021).

Many companies have used AI and gained a lot of information on customer behaviour. In any future pandemics AI can use systems such as 'robotic process automation' to handle aspects of customer activity. In the pandemic healthcare companies have used AI to plan for shortages of personal protective equipment for example, and patients have adopted AI-based apps for diagnosis and treatment of conditions that are not life threatening. Much of this is to be retained after the pandemic.

Technological development and globalisation bring about a new economy related to sustainability and social change (Popescu 2022). Coronavirus has bought about economic modifications globally that require adjustments in business models which require understanding to survive into the future.

Organisations during COVID-19 knew they had to accelerate practices that would have naturally occurred in the future. Effective e-leadership and a promotion of adaptability show that teleworking provides a significant opportunity. It can be advantageous for companies to having employees work remotely. In this work style organisations need to be less hierarchical and need to establish more trust with workers, using virtual teams to meet goals and provide satisfying work environments (Contreras, Baykal and Abid 2020).

One solution proposed during coronavirus was using robots in healthcare. There had been a high death rate of health workers from infection. Having a shortage of personal protective equipment was a major problem. Due to workload healthcare workers could not keep up with the pace of work (Zemmar, Lozano and Nelson 2020). Robots reduce staff/patient contact and work at maximum capacity. Robotic systems can have a place post-pandemic by assisting surgeons to make surgery safer, reducing time and cost. Telesurgery can also overcome expensive transport for health services to remote regions.

The appropriate use of technology including virtual peer support and new technology during COVID-19 could end up being beneficial post-pandemic. The 'peer specialist role' and its challenges during COVID-19 have been investigated in order to adapt to new service provision models. A new service delivery model, beyond coronavirus, provides opportunities for peers to develop services, their careers and allow more flexible work. Utilising virtual peer support and increasing access to technology for peers and those services worked best (Lodge et al. 2023).

Effects on people's lives

There have been varying effects of the pandemic on the lives of individuals and groups. Much of this has been due to established inequities in society.

Soga et al. (2021) argue during coronavirus and especially lockdown there have been major changes to lifestyle. This and a focus on changes on environments can lead to changes in peoples' interactions with nature. They suggest there are different opportunities, capabilities and motivation. The impact of coronavirus on lifestyle may last for years according to Soga et al. (2021).

They cite increased awareness of nature experiences, regular outdoor exercising and the practice of remote working all contribute to changed lifestyle. The virus has accentuated human-nature interactions in the short term which will potentially have widespread and long-term consequences. Knowledge gained through the pandemic could be a preparation for the future in dealing with health-related demands from addressing health-demands on greenspace, preventing negative aspects of human–nature interactions and addressing 'human–wildlife conflicts' in suburban and regional areas.

'In Denmark and Australia, the initial crisis (of COVID-19) put societies in lockdown and forced schools to digitise all educational activities. While the logistics of online teaching and learning were of great concern, there was sporadic attention given to young people's thoughts, feelings and experiences' (Rasmussen et al. 2023). An open text-based survey was conducted with over 400 students aged 15–19 years from both countries. There was also an analysis of school artefacts. The schools focussed on 'lost learning' but there was also a focus on well-being. However, young people also express concerns about aspirations and imaginings for the future. The researchers (2023) were interested in what young people said during school lockdowns and how they see the world after the pandemic. Young people were flexible but worried and frustrated for the future. They wanted contact with others, but it would risk catching the virus. However, 'the pandemic provided new ways to engage with and comprehend the world, especially in terms of climate consciousness and the meaning of life. The pandemic challenged young people to imagine other futures for the world as a whole and consequently also for themselves' (Rasmussen et al. 2023). Their critical awareness increased about how they wanted to live. The researchers dubbed them the pandemic generation, and they may want better lives than that presented to them by their elders. They wanted action, not disinterest from government, and leadership internationally in climate change for example. They wanted to live in the moment, show maturity and make mindful choices. They represent a desire for achievable futures.

A medical doctor expressed concerns about how COVID-19 affected the mental health of doctors. However, in general she says they have shown remarkable resilience. Some doctors on the frontline report having more control and connectivity with colleagues. Annual appraisals and revalidations were paused. Healthcare staff globally are being thanked for their dedication during the pandemic (Gerada 2020). However, burnout (related to being undervalued) needs to be addressed. Given a return to normality lessons from COVID-19 can be learned by the medical profession.

There are over 100 symptoms relating to COVID-19 infection (Raunkiaer et al. 2023). Shortness of breath, fatigue and cognitive influences amongst the most frequent. Longer term effects are cognitive function, fatigue, memory and concentration problems affecting everyday life and work. Raunkiaer at al. (2023) undertook a phenomenological study of people with COVID-19 symptoms and participating in a rehabilitation programme. All participants found their everyday function and work were impaired. The programme gave a vocabulary and a view of being ill and not being the same person as before COVID-19. As a result of engaging in the rehabilitation programme daily routines changed and times were set aside for mindfulness exercises and rest, and to explain the changes to family. The programme also helped set limits on workload.

A longitudinal study in Italy examined the nature of value change in different times of COVID-19. Data was initially collected by end July 2020 (Wave 1) when the virus was steadily retreating, and then in in November 2020 (Wave 2) when there was a rapid return of the virus (Vecchione and Lucidi 2022). Between Wave's 1 and 2 there was no change in 'self-enhancement, self-transcendence, conservation,' and being open to change. However economic position was related to a change in values of conservation. This meant that respondents whose income was less by Wave 2 increased their identification with self-enhancement, self-transcendence and conservation compared to those whose income remained the same. This shows the importance of income in shaping values.

Butterworth et al. (2022) found lockdowns were related to a small decrease in Australians' mental health. The effects were different for groups and followed existing inequalities in mental health. The impact of moves such as lockdowns needs further investigation. Many countries are now finding the deficits in mental health from actions during coronavirus are needing to be planned for in appropriate ways in moving beyond coronavirus.

According to Kuipers and Wolbers (2022) if anything good for the future comes out of the pandemic it is the opportunity to do comparative investigations of crisis governance. Aspects of crisis management that are important can be tried and tested under a range of conditions.

Conclusion

COVID-19 has had a range of effects on individuals, groups, communities and countries. An overriding theme has been the lines of inequality that have reflected disadvantage in virus effects and its management individually and nation-wide. Some countries put economic goals and priorities at the forefront (such as Brazil and the US). Some increased welfare, where previously there was little, and others increased an already generous welfare scheme (e.g. Nordic countries).

Inter-government cooperation was essential in closing borders and offering protection from infection. This level of cooperation is needed in the event of future pandemics and in the pursuit of global challenges such as global warming/climate change. However, the ability to prepare and protect in the future is more difficult with the unbridled pursuit of neoliberalism.

Part III

Changing impact on globalisation due to COVID-19

9 COVID-19 and climate change

This chapter starts by looking at the United Nations agreements on climate change. Further, there is a consideration of the effects of climate change on coronavirus disease-19 (COVID-19) and of the virus on climate change. Each makes an impact. Theoretical perspectives for understanding climate change are discussed. Lessons learned from both COVID-19 and climate change are a way of looking to the future, while aspects of governance and a focus on environmental justice are considered.

Public health is interested in how climate change and the pandemic intersect. Concerns about global warming, later referred to as climate change by Ronald Regan in the US (which has less severe connotations), have been expressed across the world for some decades. Despite planning at a global level to reduce emissions there has not been significant agreement until recently with most countries supporting major planned reductions (note UN 2023a). The consequences of global warming are extreme weather events and poorer countries are likely to bear the consequences. Global warming/climate change is one of the single most critical issues of our time.

International levels of agreement on emissions

Based on the Paris Agreement the overarching goal of mitigating against climate change is to hold 'the increase in the global average temperature to well below 2°C above pre-industrial levels' and pursue efforts 'to limit the temperature increase to 1.5°C above pre-industrial levels' (UN 2023a). However, global leaders have recently agreed to accept to limit global warming to 1.5°C by the end of the century. The reason is due to the UN's *Intergovernmental Panel on Climate Change (IPCC)* showing that crossing the 1.5°C level risks a far more severe impact on the effects of climate change. These include more regular heatwaves, droughts and rain. To limit global warming to 1.5°C, greenhouse gas emissions must peak before 2025 and reduce 43 per cent by 2030.

A report by Boehm and Schumer (2023) argues the level of global warming has already reached 1.1°C. On March 20, 2023, the final instalment of the Intergovernmental Panel on Climate Change's (IPCC) Sixth Assessment

DOI: 10.4324/9781003449423-12

Report (AR6) was released based on eight years of research. It reported 'already, with 1.1 degrees C (2 degrees F) of global temperature rise, changes to the climate system that are unparalleled over centuries to millennia are now occurring. in every region of the world, from rising sea levels to more extreme weather events to rapidly disappearing sea ice' (Boehm and Schumer 2023). Increased warming will multiply the effects of these changes. Every 0.5°C (0.9°F) of rising global temperature will cause discernible frequency and severity of heat extremes, regional drought and heavy rainfall. Heatwaves will occur 4.1 times more often. Adverse climate effects are more extreme than first thought. Half the world's population have scarce water at least one month per year. Higher temperatures are spreading diseases such as malaria, Lyme disease and West Nile virus.

The Paris agreement, established on November 4, 2016, has 195 members of the United Nations Framework Convention on Climate Change as parties to the agreement. Four states have not agreed. The US left in 2020 but rejoined under Joe Biden in 2021.

UN Climate Action (UN 2023b) states that '(g)oal 13 calls for urgent action to combat climate change and its impacts. It is intrinsically linked to all 16 of the other Goals of the 2030 Agenda for Sustainable Development. To address climate change, countries adopted the Paris Agreement to limit global temperature rise to well below 2 degrees Celsius.' If there is no action, temperatures will rise to more than '3 degrees Celsius this century' with some areas of the world expected to warm even more. The most vulnerable and poorest will be affected greatly. Glaciers are melting, and sea levels are rising. Effects of climate change are droughts and floods, displacing millions and bringing hunger and poverty. Access to basic services will be difficult or not possible and inequities will grow. About 700 million people may be displaced by drought alone by 2030 (UN 2023b). 2015 to 2021 were the warmest seven years on record. As of September 2023, countries were not on track to meet their targets of the Paris Agreement even though in many cases these were not stringent (Maizland 2023).

Effects of climate change on COVID-19

Climate risks can influence the experience of COVID-19. *The Lancet* (Ford et al. 2022) points out wind, humidity and temperature affect the virus transmission in ways not readily understood. Other factors appear more important. However, extremes of climate have influenced exposure to disease, emergency responses and resilience to several stressors. Climate change over the long term has increased virus risk for socio-economically vulnerable groups, including those of race and colour. These groups may face challenges to resilience, livelihoods and collapsing health systems. This can occur when people are living in areas subject to the extremes of climate change. Those exposed need public health support, emergency management, preparation in case of disasters and humanitarian support.

Effects of COVID-19 on global emissions

The OECD has identified long-term effects of COVID-19 on environment. 'There have been economic "shocks" to the environment, including to green-house gas emissions, emissions of air pollutants, the use of raw materials and land use change expected to be up to 2040' (OECD 2021c). During the pandemic environmental pressure reductions were significant (Hall-Quinlan et al. 2023; Xu et al. 2023). For example, changes in air quality in the US due to vehicular traffic significantly decreased during pandemic slowdowns (Persis and Ben Amar 2023). Methane production diminished due to the slow-down of oil, gas and refinery production (Thorpe et al. 2023). In addition, reduced traffic and energy production led to diminished carbon emissions in the US (Hwang and Papuga 2023) with emissions decreasing during lock-down in China (Liang et al. 2023). In another Chinese study by Gao et al. (2023) air pollution nationally improved in 2020 more so than through pollution control measures over the previous five years (note Yao et al. 2023). However, with an economy in recovery mode emissions are expected to increase to pre-COVID rates. There are predictions of a possible permanent 'downward impact on the levels of environmental pressures of 1–3% with a greater effect for pressures associated with economic activities that are capital intensive' (OECD 2021c).

Diffenbaugh (2022) reports both positive and negative impacts of corona-virus on environments. There have been clearer skies and wildlife returning to vacant areas. Yet benefits were temporary, and the extensive health and economic effects derived will reduce with increased emissions, created risk for many ecosystems. One question is can the lessons learned by COVID-19 be applied to the development of a newer green industry? Issues of governance, as well as control of borders, have been important during the pandemic. Governments' use of economic measures including increased welfare to support people dealing with the consequences of the pandemic have been effective. The belief in science with the pandemic is much greater than in relation to the environment and climate.

Theoretical perspectives on climate change

What is missing in the climate debate, according to Beck (2010) is the sociological perspective. Environment is more than about things. According to Beck (2015, 75) 'climate change is one of the most salient issues that peoples and governments across the world are facing – but does it have the potential to alter the social and political order of the world?' His response is yes, but beyond imagination. Beck referred to emancipatory catastrophism, referring to 'the imagination of a cosmopolitan horizon of global climate risk and oriented to changing the mode of operation of modern society toward coping with cosmopolitan climate' (Asayama 2015, 90). Asayama, critiqued Beck and posits 'apocalyptic catastrophism.'

This refers to geoengineering climate change and can be borne out by a culture of fear and catastrophe about climate and where it is heading. Walker (2021) refers to Beck's *Emancipatory Catastrophism* where he looks at how necessary it is to learn from disasters and utilise new thinking. It is insufficient to think of national borders, but worldwide, as human survival is the imperative. Like other global disasters, Hurricane Katrina in the US led to discussion of how world risk society must refute the neoliberal idea of the minimal state. This has led to more discussion of the role of the state (Beck 2006a). McBride (2016) claims it was 'reflexive re-development' based on Beck's idea, rather than disaster capitalism that restored New Orleans' racial, class and caste structures after the disaster. Walker (2021) argues Beck's position on the transformative nature in relation to lessons learned from disasters did not take place. New Orleans has still radical differences in equality and income on racial lines. Learning from disasters, as Beck suggested, is not automatic.

Hulme (2010) supports Beck's (2006b) idea of 'cosmopolitanism' and how it makes sense of sociopsychological elements of climate change: this perspective is the best way of understanding people globally. It refers to going beyond the political and philosophical to the social sciences (Beck and Grande 2012). Everyone is entitled to respect. However, Leahy (2013) disputes the claim that cosmopolitanism can bring about a paradigm change. Fiji and Pacific Islands are suffering some major effects of climate change through rising sea levels. If there is not a paradigm change then this will just further the trajectory of neoliberal globalisation.

Beck (2016) maintains that much of the climate change debate has been on whether it is real, and what can be done to address it. Looking at solutions makes it a factor of metamorphosis. Beck posits that the old establishment is falling away and a new one is emerging. China's forestation programme which has been going over decades as an eco-civilisation has parallels with Beck's metamorphosis as a transformation of a world view. The major transformations across the world needed for climate change require a 'radical reorientation of practices and perceptions' held by all proponents (Weins et al. 2023). This is when the natural and socio-political coincide. Bort and Kieser (2023) argue that asceticism has been behind several social and individual transformations. Reflecting on the work of Beck, asceticism might help people deal with climate change. It can be the impetus for igniting action for collective change.

The pandemic is a tragedy that showed some of the disintegrative aspects of Beck's risk society at a global level but conveyed what can be achieved globally with positives such as coordination, cooperation and solidarity. In relation to Beck's reflexive society theory Posocco and Watson (2023) argue that with threats larger than coronavirus such as climate change, future pandemics or wars, it is necessary to develop a new global order. Beck's concept of risk shows adaptation and insecurity as part of Fijian discourse on climate change, but less so with New Zealanders (Zaman and Das 2020).

There are problems with climate change in that it is unjust (O'Sullivan, Omukuti and Ryder 2023). Severe climate change has irreversible effects. Even without further warming irreparable damage has already occurred in some areas. Global North countries have contributed the most carbon emissions and have greater capacity to minimise emissions and adapt to climate change effects. Meanwhile, those of the Global South suffer a contrasting spread of climate harms even though they contribute minimally to global emissions (O'Sullivan et al. 2023). Global North is dominated by neoliberal, market-based approaches. The unequal relationship between the North and South is based on postcolonial lines with terms such as 'slow violence' being appropriate. Albert (2023) discusses climate emergency writers who claim action beyond normal politics is needed to meet the targets of the Paris agreement. Critics argue it could lead to suspensions of democratic rules and norms. He (2023) argues climate emergency is possible to enable the 'extraordinary politics of democracy.'

Learning from COVID-19 and climate change

Many of the lessons learned from the pandemic are applicable to climate change (Manzanedo and Manning 2020). For example, wealthier nations compared to vulnerable communities can afford to fortify against climate change. With both COVID-19 and climate change their impacts are not equally distributed. The pandemic has required global cooperation on an unparalleled scale, a situation required for tackling climate change. However, a striking difference between the two emergencies is COVID-19 can be dealt with in the short term, while climate change occurs over the long-term. Jiang et al. (2021) argue that COVID-19's effects on environment, healthcare and energy are essential for planning for the future. This is if we are to use successful models for dealing with future emergencies. There are also mutual effects of COVID-19 and climate change, on work and risk of accidents. Santurtún and Shaman (2023) have pointed out that climate change affects some jobs physically (e.g. increased heat) and psychologically. The pandemic has increased stress at work, particularly in not being able to interact satisfactorily with co-workers. Strain at work can increase the risk of accidents.

Climate change and coronavirus share global problems that need rapid government intervention. This will create losers but must be based on societal consensus and be decisive (Klenert et al. 2020). COVID-19 and climate change have similar barriers to effective action. That action can learn from the pandemic: the co-workers identify five lessons. Early action in a crisis is difficult and costly; underestimating damage affects support, and support from the public is essential for initial action; inequality can be extended by the threat and by policies to counteract it, constraining policy making; multiple international collaborations are required; and normative standpoints and effective modes of communication are needed to guard against misinformation. Klenert et al. (2020) argue that effective climate change approaches can be based on government processes applied during the pandemic. Walker (2021) presents the context of risk of climate change and the numerous challenges it poses.

Based on a media analysis during COVID-19 there were six lessons for climate change by Perkins et al. (2021). These included reducing fossil fuel consumption and emissions, the effect of a late response, the need for sustainability, rugged individualism limitations, belief in science and accommodating large change. As with the pandemic, people's health needs to be tied to a belief in government action on the climate change crisis.

There were models developed to simulate disease spread of COVID-19, limiting its impact, and there was the rapid approval of vaccines which represented a level of great cooperation between health authorities and the scientific community. According to Watson, Kundzewicz and Borrell-Damián. (2022), the previous fastest time to produce an effective vaccine comparable to one for COVID-19 was four years. Scientists have improved knowledge on loss of biodiversity and climate change and identified the corrective action needed, both short and long term. However, governments have been slow to act. 'There is no shortage of knowledge – just a shortage of political will to act in a responsible manner, and for developed countries to assist developing countries with financial and technical aid' (Watson et al. 2022, 2). As governments ignore information and advice many look to short-term politically based decisions and actions. Near term economic decisions or voter support came first for some governments. New Zealand and Australia had strong and effective programmes for COVID-19. In European countries mitigating the virus spread differed markedly. With climate change there is a comparable situation where some governments are taking corrective measures (such as in the UK and EU) which have a strong state capacity, an expert scientific community, leadership and trusting and knowledgeable populations. However, some governments with this capacity are focussed on short-term economic growth and are having large political divisions. The pursuit of neoliberalism creates problems.

According to Wahaj, Alam and Al-Amin (2022), there are similarities in some issues for both COVID-19 and climate change. Advances in technology have left vulnerable people behind and have harmed them through systemic inequalities. Dealing with coronavirus and climate change requires a whole of community approach.

Ruiu, Ragnedda and Ruiu (2020) argue that early in the pandemic the virus required a global mobilisation, but there is no similar sense of urgency about climate change. Public perception and action to tackle the problem are affected by the way they are communicated to the community. The immediate threat to life with coronavirus makes restrictions like lockdowns acceptable. However, even though there is scientific proof and media exposure of the effects of climate change such serious restrictions are untenable. Just as vaccine developments reduced the need for strict containment measures, with climate change there has not been a similar game changer and so protecting vulnerable ecosystems and communities is a way off. Sense of urgency affects interventions at the local and global level.

United Nations (UN 2021) reported reduced environmental overseeing by governments since COVID-19 began and some multilateral climate change negotiations have been postponed. However vehicular traffic decreased and there was better air quality, and reduced emissions during coronavirus. There have been effective education programmes in relation to the pandemic that can point to ways to educating about climate change. The pandemic has affected everyone, however there are varying degrees, speed and extent to which governments have had to implement top-down, unwelcomed measures. These can act as lessons in dealing with climate change. (UN 2021). When the pandemic and climate change occur together it accelerates the problems with each. It could, for example, lead to vulnerable urban populations migrating to rural regions creating increased land use and pressure which could compound climate-related problems.

Some additional parallels are drawn between the coronavirus and meeting the challenges of climate change. The focus has been on utilising styles of governance and have changed due to the impact of the COVID emergency. Bicchieri et al. (2021) report that with COVID-19, comparing compliance and belief in science to a belief in government, that compliance was greater with a belief in science. The question remains, can a belief in science at the political and decision-making level underscore the application to legislate for containing climate change?

Fuentes et al. (2020) proposed the idea that COVID-19 and climate change have similar trajectories both being global phenomena. They looked at similarities between COVID-19 and climate change, and the extent to which the virus presents examples that can help in managing climate change. They argue that both are global 'bads' and focussing on both will have a substantial social and economic cost. During coronavirus there has been international governance, essential for dealing with climate change. The virus has shown how communities are vulnerable to crises (Fuentes et al. 2020). Appropriate policy and planning need integrated approaches. This should focus on the interconnection of sustainability components and the strategies required for overall benefits. These are important governance lessons that can aid in effectively dealing with climate change globally, as well as at the national and community level. Newell and Dale (2020) argue that death from air pollution occurs more often than from COVID-19, but it is not so urgent or dramatic. Changing energy systems requires unprecedented global effort. Local action is required but national and international bodies need to ensure that climate strategies, policies and action are coordinated.

Governance for climate change

There are a number of approaches to governance for climate change. Some novel ones have been suggested by researchers. Due to the nature of global climate change its governance requires imagination, earlier referred to by

Beck (2015). It opens the possibility for reframing the relationship between the environment and humans. In this way radically different solutions can occur (Chhetri, Ghimire and Eisenhaue 2023).

The peak body for climate change is the global UN organisation which has worldwide membership and representation. It appears that much of the management of climate change happens at the local or municipal level, and if not, at the level of the city. However, the effectiveness of these strategies depends on policies and procedures at the level of the state or federal level. That is the case for funding and financing. Regional and international bodies can provide nationally binding policies.

Brown et al. (2023) reviewed the Green New Deal (GND), the UK's most ambitious environmental, social and economic programme of this century. It is implemented at local/regional levels and includes financing, green infra-structure investment and climate policy. They use a multi-governance per-spective, finding that financial system reforms of the GND and fiscal policy need to change at the national and higher levels. Most investments would be at a local level. GND needed a national programme, and the programme will be implemented at local government level if there is no national support.

Much has been written about opposition to the development of oil pipe-lines. Vogel, Johnson and Sveinsdóttir (2023) looked at the opposition to both an Enbridge's Southern Access and Dakota Access' Pipelines in the US. Landowners mobilised against the former pipeline, but not the latter, despite opposition to both. With the Enbridge's pipeline it was possible to contest it on economic grounds, leading to resistance: this was not the case for the Da-kota pipeline. The response of Illinois (US) landowners to the Dakota pipe-line was based on socio-economic historical regulator factors and citizens felt they had no real agency to affect pipeline construction. Vogel et al. (2023) argue this represents internalising 'neoliberal logics' which makes citizens' normalise market-based logic: they reasoned that the pipeline has a non-economic effect. Landowners did not have a regulatory resource to argue non-economic complaints as opposition to the pipeline and could not rise above economic attachments to their land. They asserted control by trying to maximise gains from their ceded property. It is a case where state regulations and procedures either help or hinder social mobilisation.

According to Brink and Wamsler (2018) the engagement of citizens on cli-mate change is becoming more important in policy formulation and research. While municipality involvement is vital, citizens have a legal responsibility to protect their property. Their outcomes from extreme weather events af-fect personal and public safety. Citizen participation can affect fairness and acceptability of adaptation by the public. In Sweden municipalities are the closest government bodies to citizens and despite this their relationship in terms of climate change has received little attention. The research by Brink and Wamsler (2018) has shown the potential of involving citizens in policy and research: municipalities seldom plan to include citizens in climate change adaptation. This is despite the more citizens know about climate change can lead to collective solutions. Mechanisms and structures for learning about climate change are not entirely evident. There are four issues involved in citizen engagement. Firstly, citizens need to have awareness of responsibilities and options before a hazard strikes. Secondly, a wider range of citizens need to be engaged to promote equity of inclusion. Then, nature-based solutions are needed to link with broader social change. Finally, better municipal interdepartmental coordination is required.

Some time ago urgency was expressed on strategies for dealing with climate change. Baird, Plummer and Bodin (2016) citing the need for collaboration in governance approaches stressed adaptive co-management. Their study in Canada used a network perspective to examine social relationships and a collaborative initiative to address the problem. They found that good network structures and relationships were not enough to develop an adaptive co-management process. On its own it may not be enough for dealing with climate change.

Other studies have addressed the issue of governance in dealing with the causes and consequences of climate change. For example, Cattivelli (2023) argues despite European concerns, specific guidelines are not yet in place for macro-regional level governance for climate change. Macro-regions consist of multiple regions with some shared characteristics. Currently larger-scale approaches do not fully consider government or territorial issues at regional levels, or the needs of neighbours.

Zimmermann et al. (2023b) present potential solutions to extensive flooding in India. Disaster risk reduction and climate change adaptation are both needed to be managed locally, at the municipal and neighbourhood level. Actors at that level are often overlooked. In another study on municipal level governance Yang et al. (2023) reviewed the effects of increasing migration in Ontario, Canada. Higher numbers of migrants are related to poorer environmental outcomes. There needs to be more municipal services and investment in environment as a result. In France, effects of climate change in river systems utilise a balance of bottom-up and top-down governance (Aubin et al. 2019). Local water authorities and water commissions are the main proponents with a crucial role in climate change management.

Óvári, Kovács and Farkas (2023) cite increasing knowledge of environment issues and the European Green Deal are behind increasing attention on climate change in Hungarian cities. The co-workers found the 'mandated climate planning process' and being dependent on EU funding had negative effects on climate-focussed approaches. Cities in urban areas are becoming more the focus of climate action.

Lessons for climate change from the governance of COVID-19

Given that the pandemic and climate change are two of the most major events the lessons learned on governance are important for the future. There were some important things that occurred out of managing and mitigating COVID-19.

Ryner (2023) argues the EU COVID-19 Recovery Plan and Green Deal are hard to depoliticise in European neoliberal governance. The framework of the Energy Union promoted the EU's climate targets' integration into the energy transition policy of the EU before the European Green Deal. The EU's COVID-19 response made for strong policy and financial bases to enable the green transition (Crnčec, Penca and Lovec 2023). Scognamiglio et al. (2023) report that public sector organisations worked with others to create robust governance during COVID-19. The process of co-creation is where two or more actors try to solve a problem. This is done through exchanging competencies, knowledge, resources and ideas enhancing public value and strategies, and frameworks for finding new solutions. Rana and Fleischman (2023) report that forest bureaucrats in India did not always handle COVID-19 well. Some officers at this level did not control or manage offences or livelihoods. Outdated laws and a lack of professionalism contributed. In Japan effective governance by the government was lacking which hindered the use of digital technologies during COVID-19 (Kodama 2023).

Currently, there are global disruptions that need coordinated responses by business and other social agencies, across local, national and international sectors. International governance used with COVID-19 is a requirement for dealing with climate change. The pandemic focussed on vulnerabilities in communities. Sustainability issues are interconnected. Some argue that coronavirus responses needed to focus on climate risks (especially on extremes), preparing for disasters and looking at the humanitarian consequences.

Many of the lessons learned by COVID-19 can be translated and applied to the development of a newer 'green' industry. Governments have used economic measures including increased welfare to support people dealing with the economic and social consequences of the pandemic. There are discussions on compensating poorer nations affected by climate change (although in July 2023 the US ruled this possibility out). However, in November 2023 it was announced that Australia would provide some climate relief for Tuvalu, comprising 11 islands in the mid-Pacific (Frost 2023). Due to rising sea levels caused by climate change Australia agreed to 280 citizens of Tuvalu out of a total of 11,200 to migrate to Australia. This is not a large step but nonetheless a concession to a country being affected by climate change.

Ulrich Beck's work on global risk and climate change and other sociological perspectives are important to understanding that there should not be a repetition of colonial inequities with climate change, nor a pure reliance on neoliberalism.

Environmental justice

'Mitigating the impact of environmental disasters and climate change on vulnerable groups of people calls for an environmental justice–based approach that makes "the fair treatment and meaningful involvement of all people regardless of race, colour, national origin, or income" a top priority'

(Kapadia 2023, 12). He continues that the climate threat is real. The International Panel on Climate Change Special Report on Global Warming says a 1.5°C increase for the US will escalate environmental disasters worldwide. This will bring heat waves, more droughts, worse floods and rain, sea level increases and reduced polar ice caps. To address the lack of focus on oceans and coastal communities in the Green New Deal, Axon et al. (2023) proposed a Blue New Deal in the US. In it, environmental justice and sustainability for oceans and coastal regions are crucial to its success in enhancing its role and its management. This is a comprehensive approach to managing the environment.

Environmental justice means that the inequities exposed by COVID-19 must be guarded against in dealing with global warming/climate change. It takes political will to confront those unequal outcomes and if they are not, there will be severe global repercussions.

Conclusion

There are parallels between climate change and COVID-19. Both are global disasters, and both require global solutions. The work of Ulrich Beck on risk and the outcomes of catastrophes sheds a light on needing to consider the human side in seeking solutions to climate change. Modes of dealing with global bads can glean some support from the successes in dealing with the pandemic.

In the future pandemics can pose a threat, but the experience of dealing with COVID-19 can lead to dealing better at a global level with that threat. However, as with coronavirus, so with climate change, those who will be most affected will be the disadvantages by race, class, colour and gender. Solutions will be unbalanced and will not sustain the whole of the world unless these inequities are dealt with.

10 Growth of the green industry, labour and the labour process

This chapter points out that becoming resource efficient and having a low carbon economy needs changes in production in several areas. Energy, waste management and agriculture use a lot of resources and have elevated levels of emissions (ILO 2018). Moving to greener jobs is directly and indirectly related to these sectors. Resource efficiency needs to increase. In recent times in the US 19.4 per cent of employees could work in the green economy (this would also include indirect green jobs), without the need for substantial changes in knowledge or skills. Further, the pandemic is shown to affect the green economy, and contributions of greenness to sustaining health during the pandemic are discussed.

The International Labour Organisation (ILO 2023a) reports that we need to transition to a carbon- and resource-efficient economy. 'Climate change and environmental degradation are already disrupting millions of jobs and livelihoods. Yet countless opportunities lie ahead to boost the economy and improve the quality of working lives. Implementing the Paris Agreement on Climate Change could create a net gain of 18 million jobs by 2030' (ILO 2023a). Government, employers and employees are encouraged to develop a sustainable environment process and create reasonable jobs. 'Green jobs are defined as economically viable employment that reduces environmental impacts to sustainable levels' (ILO 2023a). This encompasses jobs that restore and promote ecosystems and biodiversity and reduce energy use, materials and resources. These jobs reduce carbon in the economy and avoid or use less waste and pollution.

Currently, renewables in terms of electricity worldwide look to be 45 per cent in 2030, and with the right support electric cars and the building sector adaptions would increase. China is leading in sales of electric vehicles (EVs) and sustainable and energy efficient construction is increasing. Both areas provide growth in employment and the need to learn new skills. If recovery spending packages from the pandemic focussed on hastening the transition to low-carbon energy and improving the efficiency of energy, there could be a much-needed boost to reaching the targets of the Paris Agreement. Dafnomilis et al. (2022) maintain that even though there has been a significant financial recovery for coronavirus disease-19 (COVID-19) there is only a low

DOI: 10.4324/9781003449423-13

proportion allocated to green recovery. If one per cent of worldwide Gross Domestic Product (GDP) were for financially supporting measures to emissions for three years, this could lead to 10.5–15.5-per cent reduction in CO_2 emissions by 2030. This is below the figure estimated before COVID-19.

Conti et al. (2018) discuss the integration of the European Union (EU)'s renewable energy sources. Renewable energy sources and technologies have been prominent in the EU member states since the late 1980s: they address environmental and economic concerns. They are a means of diversifying energy supply and create less dependence on imported fossil fuels. There will be new work and skills created in areas that are progressive and have potential 'high growth.' Many other regions have also made important inroads in the development of a green economy.

Ecological risk challenges the development of modern society. Bardsley and Knierim (2020) maintain that Beck (1992) and Beck, Giddens and Lash (1994) created intractable risks in response to development, in the idea of an alternative reflexive modernity. This is where many paths exist to sustainable development. There is risk at all levels incorporating nature and allowing an 'ecological dialect.' Bardsley and Knierim (2020) argue that Australian agriculture demonstrates there is risk taking a path that is inappropriate. Agricultural communities need to respond to risk with state-of-the art research, training and policymaking. Key ecological principles need to be incorporated.

Globalisation and green industry

The idea of a green economy goes back to the early 1970s (Chen et al. 2023). In 2009 it gained importance when the global community started to pursue 'sustainable policies' in relation to CO_2 emissions and economic growth. Brazil, Russia, South Africa and especially India and China, following Europe and North America, moved towards increasing their share of renewable energy sources. The development of green industries is at the background to changing labour forces worldwide. Some say it will require large levels of upskilling while others see only moderate changes. Green growth involves green technological innovations to achieve green production as well as green supply chains. Green growth can save energy, reduce emissions and control damage to the environment. To achieve this and the efficiency of production, there is green technological innovation. Patents and environmental innovation estimates have been positive in the long term, showing that technologies are helping with green growth in several countries. A positive financial globalisation leads to green growth in these economies, with a greater focus on research and development needed.

Zhang et al. (2023b) maintain globalisation has had major environmental effects, regionally and internationally. With neoliberalism and reliance on the market there are fewer checks on business activities. Business innovation and advancement however affect pollution and air quality. Financial growth can lead to degradation of the environment, but several studies show a positive effect.

The researchers (2023b) maintain there should be private environmental projects because they lead to financial development and at the same time reduce pollution. In the Middle East and North African countries energy consumption and pollution need attention. These include Saudi Arabia and Israel as high-income countries, Iran and Jordan as middle income and Tunisia and Egypt as lower income countries. Solar, biofuel, wind and thermal materials all need attention. Zhang et al. (2023b) found that globalised developments in the financial sector had a strong effect on ecological quality. Foreign investment in these countries may create problems if CO_2 emissions are not controlled such as in extraction industries. The environmental problems are greater with increased levels of investment. Neoliberal globalisation in these countries faces the same obstacles as in developed countries of increasing emissions and being ecologically harmful. Examples of these are in mining and energy industries. Few studies have shown financial developments having positive effects and leading to reducing environmental discharge. Increasing the use of energy will bring about harmful emissions. Also, more information and access to appropriate technologies through foreign investors is needed. Using 1971–2015 figures, globalisation and financial development needs improvement while foreign direct investment is needed within environmental guidelines. Middle East and North African governments need to develop renewable energy.

According to Ahmad and Satrovic (2023), environmental taxation has a powerful effect in reducing global emissions. Yet they maintain that the ecological benefits of green taxes in transport have been mostly overlooked. The co-workers looked at Group of Seven (G7) countries between 1994–2016 and found transport sector taxes have a neutral influence in the short term but provided ecological stability long term. It was the same effect for ecological sustainability in the long run but being neutral in the short run. For these countries for higher economic growth, ecological recovery occurred in the long run. Transport sector taxes can strongly diminish emissions and provide ecological quality. With globalisation, green investment and trading in environmentally beneficial products can lead to sustainable development.

The extractive industry uses a huge amount of energy: it contributes enormously to greenhouse gas emissions. By 2020, worldwide extractive industry emissions were 7.7 billion tons of CO_2 or 15 per cent of the global anthropogenic emissions (with some exclusions). The greatest emitter was China. Natural resources have been raw materials for economic development – mineral resources. This has risen globally in recent years. China produces 19 per cent of energy and consumes 24 per cent of global energy. Extractive industries have major adverse environmental effects. Mineral extraction has led to deteriorating ecosystems, pollution of the environment, landscape damage, 'ecological disasters' and health problems. There has been less attention paid to its impact on climate change (Zheng et al. 2023). Economic recovery from COVID-19 poses specific challenges for future emissions. China's GDP growth reduced to 2.3 per cent in 2020 but increased to 8.1 per cent in 2021.

Extraction factors are a major component of emissions. Natural resource extraction and processing account for around a half of 'global greenhouse emissions.' Activities involved include ore mining and extraction, smelting and refining. Extractive activities are likely to increase in the future affecting emissions and natural degradation, due to mining of low-grade ores from fragile sites. Most deposits of ore have already been depleted. The most critical path for reducing emissions is to focus on reducing coal mining.

'Given the challenges posed by the climate crisis, human over-population and food insecurity, the future of agri-food production relies on indoor, vertical, smart and high-tech automation in hitherto unimaginable scenarios' (Fradejas-García, Molina and Lubbers 2023, 1). What is referred to as the 'sea of plastic' is a semi-desert area of 450 km^2 in Almería, Spain. Intensive farming covered by plastic is located there. In an agro-industrial area it is called 'Europe's farm,' and it produces out-of-season vegetables for millions of Europeans. It is connected to the regime controlled by multinational companies and agribusiness capital. This is a globalised arrangement in an agro-industrial district: grassroots activity is important here. There are 10,000 Spanish farmers who own the land. They have positive outcomes from a network of local companies and maintain control over production and marketing. Labour is cheap, provided by 50,000 workers primarily immigrants working precariously and being exploited. They come from eastern Europe and Africa. In the 2000s several Romanians ran businesses in greenhouse auxiliary companies such as in repairs and building of greenhouses. They went on to develop highly successful agri-food ventures.

Labour, labour process and green jobs

Before COVID-19 there was globalisation, technological change and automation, and the creation of green industries. This signalled a divide where cities benefit from these changes. Other regions did not and faced disadvantage. Sixty-one per cent of people in 28 countries in 2015 felt the rate of change with technology was too fast. In 2020 in the US 13 per cent of people were in jobs that did not exist in 1970 (OECD 2020c). In addition, due to automation, rural regions in the US have been at risk of large job losses. Eighteen per cent of jobs in Organisation for Economic Cooperation and Development (OEDC) countries are green. The uptake and growth of these industries depends on skill availability. Women are under-represented in green jobs accounting for 28 per cent of jobs. The move to greenness requires more education. COVID-19 progresses trends such as urbanisation, and governments need to address the ramifications. Skilled labour markets have grown over recent decades and technology has led to polarised jobs.

There are threats to the labour market in moving to a green economy. There is potential exploitation of third-world workers in pursuing base products for sustainable industries of the first world (note the experience of Congolese workers in mining cobalt discussed later in this chapter, Zeuner 2018).

In developed countries such as the US there are regulations enacted stipulating that a high proportion of electric cars must be sold by 2030 (Silva, Carley and Konisky 2023), requiring skills training of the workforces. Some claim there will be large skills changes, especially with automation skill updating requiring training. Others claim some work will be at a low skills level, with some misleading job opportunities (Castellini 2019). While unions have been under pressure for the past two decades they are needed to protect labour with the burgeoning economy of green jobs (Goods 2011). Concerns in the US have been expressed by automobile workers as well as by workers in other industries facing large technological change.

Greenness can be seen as a continuum (Bowen, Kuralbayvea and Lipoe 2018). Changes in control over the job are focussed on, for example, in the mining industry where there have been large developments in automation. Green jobs may provide greater control opportunities for workers, but it depends on the extent of automation. Workers may have increases in skills and expertise which can lead to enhancing their control over their work.

Cobalt mining

The exploitation of third-world cheap labour sources for resources used in ecological products such as batteries for computers and mobile phones is an unwanted side effect of green innovation. Zeuner (2018) addresses the mining of cobalt in the Democratic Republic of Congo (DRC), for use in rechargeable lithium-ion batteries, as energy storage. The researcher outlines that decisions to include the Congolese in supply has had ramification on political stability and corruption in the DRC. Cobalt is very heat resistant and is used in storage batteries in EVs. DRC in 2017 had at least half of the global supply of cobalt.

Between 2000 and 2020 China's production of cobalt increased 78 times (Gulley 2023). Many of these producers sought cobalt from the DRC. Artisanal production (by freelance workers) was mainly either exported to China or processed by Chinese firms in DRC. Up to 79 per cent of production was carried out in the DRC. Computers, smartphones and EVs represent the future of the modern world, but the rechargeable batteries are often based on cobalt mined in the DRC by slave-like workers including children (Gross 2023). Pay is as low as 30c per hour. This cannot represent a 'clean' supply chain.

Electric vehicles

China now is the main country in the manufacture of EVs (Yang 2023). The author points out that compared to US sales of around 800,000 EVs, China sold 6.800,000 in 2022. Germany is also a major market for EVs. The Chinese experience of these vehicles has been achieved through government support including subsidies, procurement contracts, tax incentives and a number of local EV brands and developing new technologies.

In 2021 the US government announced plans to make 50 per cent of new vehicles sold in 2030 zero emissions. EVs are a major form of decarbonisation (Silva, Carley and Konisky 2023). While this is a substantial contribution, traditional automobile workers need to have their voices heard. It is not clear whether the EV industry will have non-unionised positions with temporary appointments, hourly or workers with less pay. Community members and managers are confident that the long-term agility of the automobile industry would prevail in the future. In contrast, autoworkers felt EV technology was overstated and didn't meet consumer needs. They felt their past work for the auto industry would be forgotten and felt suspicious about green energy.

Unions

Goods (2011) proposed labour organisations as central to bringing sustainability and labour together. Writing more than a decade ago he argued that labour unions are essential in an environmentally sustainable future. Ecological sustainability needs biodiversity and keeping natural capital for intergenerational equity. There are a range of jobs labelled green. According to Goods a 'treadmill of production' effect can explain how capitalist production can be ecologically destructive. To gain profits corporations need to expand production. This creates conflicts and tensions between workers' needs and interests, and environmental concerns. Political elites and the state are also involved in this treadmill. There have been concerns about the continuity of jobs amid environmental issues. 'Green capitalism' has recast the relationship between jobs and environment. Protecting the environment is cutting edge investment and opportunities. Adding to the union, jobs and environment debate Räthzel and Uzzell (2011) argue that for some time international union bodies have been involved in environment issues.

Approaches to greenness

The 'jobs-environment-dilemma' resulted from severe ecological impacts due to work. This occurred because of the 'structural constitution' of industrial society's centring on work. Society is work dependent. In modern society there is a jobs-environment dilemma, where jobs usually come first. Hoffmann and Paulsen (2020) argue that most sustainability research does not include discussions of jobs. However, it is chiefly through production that negative ecological effects occur. They (2020) introduce the concept of 'postwork,' being a critique of work and look at how 'postwork' can address established sustainability issues. Postwork involves critiques of work and of work society. It signals a transformation of industrial society and involves 'not necessarily …. abolishing work tout-court, but rather …. pointing out and questioning its relentless centrality and asking what a more desirable, free and sustainable society might look like' (Hoffmann and Paulsen 2020, 348). A critical point is that in the short term how do some citizens survive socioeconomically and sociopsychologically in this proposed radical transformation of work?

Under neoliberalism, green economies are market driven and therefore based on exploitation of labour and nature, and on their commodification. However, their proponents undertake to obscure and secure these processes (Castellini 2019). These include forming and disseminating an ideology of green labour in relation to environmentalism. In a study of green job advertisements in Canada, the ideology surrounding green work looks to select productive and motivated workers. In this study of newspaper advertisements for green jobs, the advertisers justify offering precarious or nonpaid work, and non-specialised positions. These include positions regarded outside the sphere of employment, such as, for example environmentalist activism. The researcher (2019) argues that this shows examples of how the green economy can use exploited labour.

The idea of point of production, control and emotional labour in the 'gig economy' (for example Uber) is presented by Gandini (2019). The researcher argues that labour process theory gives a pertinent perspective for understanding how labour power is transformed into a commodity. This is where a digital platform mediates demand and supply of work. Ratings and rankings are based on managerialism, that is, carried out by professional administrator and reliant on metrics. The gig economy is growing as digital technologies increase and looks to be a part of our work future where the growth and influence of ecological issues increases (note Holland, Brewster and Kouglannou 2021). The global volume of this business was $US455 bill in 2023. In the same year the number of independent workers in the US was 31.9 mill, up from 15.8 mill in 2020 (Statista 2023). Gandini (2019) continues that a labour process approach identifies that the point of production is not in a defined workplace. Further, in relation to emotional labour, it is based on feedback, rating and ranking systems utilising a techno-normative form of control. Women, when working from home, are measured through metrics by management systems and this intersects with emotional labour they are engaged in, therefore, increasing control over their homelife.

Currently agroecological production does not provide more effective systems for all agricultural production. The ILO (2022) has worked with farmers in Chaing Mai (Thailand) to develop sustainable agriculture. The skills required must be learned by workers to have successful sustainability, giving them good, transferrable skills. Some countries have not yet taken full advantage of these systems. The extent to which agroecological production systems (sustainable farming with nature) provide better conditions of work than other agricultural systems was investigated by Dumont and Baret (2017). Initially, due to political, social and economic circumstances on face value agroecological vegetable production does not offer better work experiences than conventional or organic systems. However medium-sized agroecological market gardening has the best situation, and small agroecological producers have the worst, which is in relation to all other vegetable production systems. Producers must balance inheritance issues, work orientation, career, beliefs and values and socio-cultural factors. Poor-quality equipment and manual work alone affect discomfort more than the 'degree of mechanisation,' socio-cultural heritage, beliefs and values of the producers (note employer and employee roles in green work by Montt 2018).

Green behaviour by workers contributes to environmental sustainability. It can enhance environmental protection, and backup an organisation's coping efforts with ecological pressure. Wu, Tang and Sun (2018) found green behaviour by employees in Chinese workplaces was demonstrated by pro-environmental consciousness and green psychological climate. It was the interactive effects of these two elements that formed the basis of the new generation (people being born after 1980).

How work is carried out can affect organisational and sustainable goals. A study of greenness in working conditions suggests it may result in organisational goal improvements, including sustainability. Liu et al. (2021) state that non-green labour includes long hours of work and poor protection for labour. Working hours for Chinese employees have grown enormously, surpassing even those in Japan. With the growth of new technology, protection at work needs to improve. Non-green work patterns affect health and sustainable development in organisations. Labour protection (for physical and mental health) is required for sustainable development of the workforce. Liu et al. (2021) found that institutional constraints impeded employees' requirement for green labour. However, good skills and psychological resources help protect against organisational constraints.

The uptake of labour into green jobs is more than just shifting workers. It may involve learning new skills for example, but jobs involving an uptake of technology (especially information technology) may increase their control over work. A warning, however, is there needs to be vigilance in the face of low-level jobs offerings under employment. This can lead to exploitation.

COVID-19 and the green economy

The transition to a resource-efficient and low carbon economy requires changing production methods across several sectors. Agriculture, transport, energy and waste management need to become more resourceful and have emissions reduced. These industries use many resources and can employ many workers.

COVID-19 has brought about a rethink of the social and economic models derived from neoliberal globalisation as countries have moved through coronavirus. One important priority remains: that the green economy and green industries grow. Green financing and technology impact on UN CO_2 targets. Lessons from global cooperation in COVID-19 and of governance become planning benchmarks for expanding a green economy. Socio-political factors are likely to affect this. The political decision-making processes are important, where more positive steps are occurring in sustainability policy by certain political parties and not others.

During the pandemic forces were mobilised to contain and control infection and deaths, with national and international resources fully engaged with the virus. Long-term goals such as the development of green industries had a more limited focus during this time. As part of green developments, investor confidence may have dampened.

Green bonds

COVID-19 has led to rising production costs and the reduction of economic and human resources. Green financial policies (including carbon pricing, green certificates that are transferrable, and green credit) can reduce the cost of the epidemic (Hu and Zhu 2023). Green bonds and loans are important to China's energy conservation and environmental protection business, which has high investment risk. 'As declared by the World Bank and OECD, green bonds are generally defined as a sustainable fix-income instrument, one of the most important avenues to finance environment-friendly projects' (Imran and Ahad 2023, 108). They represent investment that is sustainable long term and have become a tool for guarding against financial risks, rare disasters and climate change.

COVID-19, geopolitical risks and targets of net-zero have provided incentives as well as pressures particularly for those investing in renewable energy. It is now the biggest energy sector (Demiralay, Gencer and Kilincarslan 2023). Importantly, clean energy companies outperformed other sectors.

Energy supplies need to be decarbonised (Hanna, Xu and Victor 2020). However, during COVID-19, there was an inward turning to health, the economy and jobs. In the initial stages of coronavirus, the US, Mexico, South Africa and several other countries relaxed pollution control laws and vehicle energy efficiency standards. Transport is the greatest source of emissions in the US. Fortunately, investing in energy efficient and renewable industries can save hundreds of thousands of jobs.

There have been calls to create a more sustainable path (Chen et al. 2020). The European Commission sees green financial incentives as the basis of growth. Thorpe (2020) argues that the best way of recovering from coronavirus is through investing in green jobs. Xames, Shefa and Sarwar (2023) added that the bicycle industry could aid recovery. However, jobs at risk during COVID-19 may not be supported by the green economy. Strachan, Greig and Jones (2023) report there has been a gross underestimation of skills needed in new green jobs. One change is business groups may see Zoom or its equivalents as a preferable alternative to travel to meetings and conferences, thus, removing a reliance on fossil fuels through air travel.

Moving from coronavirus to sustainability models

A study in Pakistan looked at the effect of job insecurity during coronavirus on influencing intentions to be green entrepreneurs (Noor, Rabbani and Dastgeer 2022). Entrepreneurial passion was also measured for its effect as well as environmental knowledge and consciousness. It was important as it affected the relationship between COVID-19 and job insecurity. Being a green entrepreneur refers to having a business which is environmentally friendly, particularly in relation to coronavirus, with an orientation to hygiene and cleanliness.

Pollitt et al. (2021) showed how a green package for recovery out of COVID-19 could provide support for the world economy and labour markets nationally. This would perform better than a conventional stimulus approach and reduce global emissions by 12 per cent. Using 'car scrappage' that leads to using electric vehicles has the biggest effect on jobs and GDP. However, the reduction in emissions through meeting short-term recovery out of coronavirus and boosting sustainability in the long term is not sufficient to achieve globally 2°C and not just 1.5°C. In a study of 14 territories during COVID-19 Liu et al. (2023) found that a reduction of 6.01 per cent could be found in global carbon emissions, while export carbon emissions were virtually unaffected. Coronavirus mostly affected the energy products area. Impacts were higher in developing countries (having resource-based organisations) compared to developed countries.

COVID-19 had some positive environmental effects, but there were some negative effects for conservation and biodiversity (Sandbrook, Gómez-Baggethun and Adams 2022). The consumption of wild species by people eating or selling food increased in developing countries. In addition, economic downturn, the decline in tourism and changed donor priorities led to a financial loss for conservation organisations. Beyond the short-term impacts of COVID-19, there is a need to review national and international policies, and ways of avoiding recession. Late in the pandemic most nations have been struggling with the threat of recession. Four policy responses in relation to COVID-19 are: restoration of the previous economy, removing impediments to economic growth, undertaking a green recovery and a transformation through economic reconstruction. Each of these provide both risks and opportunities for conservation. Sandbrook et al. (2022) argue that the post-epidemic recovery approach chosen will affect biodiversity futures.

Bærenholdt and Meged (2023) examined tourism in Copenhagen to meet the challenge of climate change. They looked at a changing discourse of tourism. The Copenhagen approach was to engage with locals who had access to attractions offered to tourists. Extensions were planned for the airport to help with sustainable development. The city plans to be the tourist destination with most sustainability, despite that travellers arriving may have large emissions through air travel. Models of governance based on neoliberalism have been used in the tourist industry, which was devastated by coronavirus.

According to Robina-Ramíraz et al. (2022) the virus gave excellent lessons in sustainable governance models. They examined tourism in a region of Spain and proposed developing public/private interactions, establishing corporate values, enhancing cooperative governance models, improve local involvement in decision-making and utilising qualitative goals. Further, Pröbstl-Haider, Gugerell and Maruthaveeran (2023) discuss the effect of COVID-19 on nature and outdoor recreation-based tourism. They pose the question whether the high level of visiting forests, parks and recreation facilities will remain after the virus. There are also effects on urban management and for planning post-coronavirus. These could lead to new target groups for nature-based tourism and recreation. Cai et al. (2023) discuss further sustainable tourism as it relates to green and low carbon revitalisation.

Lisbon was given the title of the Green capital of Europe in 2020, based on its sustainability during an economic crisis. After a year COVID-19 had devastating effects (including confinement for individuals and no physical contact). However, why was Lisbon not sustainable or resilient? Job losses were high and there were supply problems as Portugal imports 70 per cent of its food. As in many parts of the world vulnerabilities were exposed. Simon (2023) argues that Urban Agriculture (UA), for example, could provide solutions to sustainability and confront some of the inequities exposed through coronavirus.

Many people were at risk of severe COVID-19 consequences. They were most likely to be affected by restrictions imposed in containing the virus. Green spaces positively influence health effects of some coronavirus restrictions (Geary et al. 2021). Urban green spaces which are publicly accessible can be an important social investment and create a balance with nature as a protection for future pandemics. Green spaces need to be enhanced and protected and to balance inequities. Lehberger, Kleih and Sparke (2021) undertook a comparison between those with and without gardens during coronavirus.

The pandemic reduced consumer confidence and contracted the economy. The airline industry reduced significantly as a result. Slower recovery due to border closures was predicted (Xuan et al. 2021). Return to travel needed government stimulus packages. In 2023 several airlines were operating as most coronavirus restrictions had been lifted. Guillen-Royo (2022) addresses how flight behaviour changed in Norway because of COVID-19. Norway has some of the highest rates of flight per capita in Europe. Keeping global warming to 1.5°C may not happen without air travel restrictions. If flight frequency stays low after the pandemic then people working in flight intensive sectors may have some sociopsychological benefits due to job security.

Other impacts of greenness

Angheluță and Badea (2018) review the role of human capital in sustainable development. Cities are involved in efforts to decrease the effects of climate change. There needs to be a focus on waste recycling and reduction and increasing the energy performance of buildings. Transport is another area for development. There can be green spaces established with public lighting using renewable energy. Written prior to COVID-19 Angheluta and Badea (2018) suggest that the vulnerability of cities may increase due to natural disasters.

Does ecological restoration (e.g., vegetation cover) influence the income gap? Based on the data collected on 290 cities in China (2007–2018), Ma, Tian and Zhang (2023) found ecological restoration reduced income inequality. However, due to social discrimination, employment opportunities and educational attainment, reducing the gap will take time. Green industry funding from local managers and the government is required, and more technical training needed for migrant workers and the poor.

Gan et al. (2023) maintain there has been little research on the impact of technology on green innovation. Between 2011 and 2019 in China the use of robots helped with green innovation, in terms of savings on labour costs and changes in human capital structure. This happened in firms with high levels of Research and Development (R&D) investment, using advanced technology and with more exacting environmental regulations. Consumer acceptance of autonomous delivery robots (ADRs) was studied by Koh and Yuen (2023) as coronavirus had utilised contactless deliveries. Consumer intention to adopt ADRs was affected by their technology and health perspectives.

Conclusion

The future is in low emissions and a sustainable economy. COVID-19 has delivered a social and economic shock to the world and brings with it a caution of how we must protect ourselves for the future. Other pandemics and the reality of climate change need attention. Green jobs in a green economy are needed for planning, policy and investment by nation states and international organisations. Socio-political factors are important. In globally sustainable, low emission goals are often overlooked in favour of short-term goals of employment and economic growth. These are important but should not overshadow longer-term sustainability goals. Much depends on the political machinations of nations and requires the political will to bring about changes.

11 Changes in local, national and global labour markets

It is argued that labour markets have been undergoing transitions during recent times. Theoretical issues, mainly based on Beck, are presented. Globalisation has had a significant impact on labour markets. Further there is discussion of local, national and international labour markets during coronavirus, and finally, the effect of the virus on migrant and refugee labour is presented.

The labour market is likely to become more skilled because of coronavirus disease-19 (COVID-19), but one sector that has diminished during the pandemic is universities. Their growth reduced due to the lack of international education, and in countries such as Australia universities were not financially supported during the pandemic. This has national implications for education and training. Those most affected by COVID-19 are younger workers, comprising many who are in casualised and precarious work. It is likely that due to COVID-19 some young people may be delayed from gaining permanent work. Many precarious workers lost their jobs during the pandemic.

Risks involved in modernity and the nature of work including precarity are relevant to understanding Ulrich Beck. Chan and Tweedie (2016) maintain that, despite criticism, Beck discusses the nature of employment insecurity. While some of Beck's claims were overstated there is evidence of increases in insecurity in specific nations, industries and worker groups. We have witnessed a steady growth of precarity (note Tweedie and Chan 2021). With the development of the 'gig' economy, deregulation has increased insecurity, or it may be work is being regulated to benefit capital. Neoliberalism has employed deregulation as a cornerstone, and this has meant the labour market has moved into a growing state of flexibility. With the market dominating, labour has become more malleable. Beck analysed novel structures of insecurity, which 'draws more nuanced links between patterns and politics of insecurity than critics of Beck's "Brazilianization" thesis typically acknowledge' (Chan and Tweedie 2016, 896). Employment insecurity is also spreading which the co-workers argue is matched by insecurity in higher level occupations.

With the knowledge of COVID-19 effects on labour markets, the world has seen the consequences of three or more decades of neoliberalism. Without

DOI: 10.4324/9781003449423-14

local, regional, state and international actions and cooperation, outcomes from neoliberalism could have been worse. Vulnerabilities in the labour market have followed historic lines with migrants, people of colour and many women historically experiencing inequity.

Labour market trends during COVID-19

Labour markets globally significantly declined in 2022. 'Emerging geopolitical tensions, the Ukraine conflict, an uneven recovery from the pandemic, and ongoing bottlenecks in supply chains have created the conditions for a stagflationary episode, the first period of simultaneously high inflation and low growth since the 1970s' (ILO 2023b). Looking at the global level there has been high inflation and jobs recovery is not complete. Globally, hours worked, and employment levels mostly have not returned to pre-COVID-19 levels. A number of countries have a significant amount of debt. Many of the employed are unable to have social protection and rights at work. Again globally, unequal labour markets exist with women and young people experiencing disadvantage. In 2022 214 million workers were living in extreme poverty. Two billion were engaged in informal jobs. Another factor is that climate change is starting to influence the labour market. It is expected the employment growth rate for 2023 is one per cent – this compares negatively to 2.3 per cent the year before. There have been no employment gains in the US, with Europe and Central Asia being strongly affected by the conflict in the Ukraine. (ILO 2023c). Decent work has implications for social justice.

Due to COVID-19 governments globally compiled lists of critical occupations and sectors so that workers could ensure relevant infrastructure, delivery of nursing and medical care and the supply of crucial goods. Essential workers had some supports (albeit not for mobile and migrant workers) so they could do their tasks, while other workers were told to isolate and reduce contact at work. Working conditions in these jobs were worse than in other jobs. COVID-19 produced labour market social inequality and job strain, particularly in critical jobs which provide medical, nursing and essential goods. Dütsch (2022) argues there are few studies investigating the working conditions for these jobs. The researcher analysed the Working Time Survey for Germany (2019). Having critical jobs made up 53.48 per cent of the sample. These were in transport and logistics, cleaning and healthcare, as well as medical care and natural science services. Workers in essential services received lower wages. Their jobs made them more likely to work near others, mostly they could not work from home and worked more atypical times. They were also more at risk of musculoskeletal injuries.

Italy was one of the hardest hit counties with the COVID-19 pandemic. In 2020 its Gross Domestic Product (GDP) had contracted by 8.9 per cent and the virus continued to be a problem despite measures such as work compensation schemes and freezing of layoffs (Cerqua and Letta 2022). The economic fallout was great and varied across regions, but not like the pattern of the Great Recession. The largest losses in employment were related to those previously vulnerable in the labour market.

There were economic costs of COVID-19 for workers, leading to health and well-being problems and a loss of earnings. If they had families and/or dependents these losses can affect the health, well-being, educational attainment and even the long-term career success of their offspring. Also, school and nursery closures may compound the problems (Hupkau et al. 2023). The labour market shock may have ramifications, in this case, well beyond coronavirus. Measured at two points in time (April 2020 and January 2021) in the UK, the co-workers looked at consequences of the shocks of the virus on economic livelihood. The biggest negative effects were where earnings dropped, and this was more evident for fathers than mothers. In April 2020 fathers were spending about half an hour per day helping with schoolwork but this decreased significantly by January 2021 as negative work events became more persistent. Household income started to diminish as did fathers' mental health.

Effects on employment and unemployment

In the US COVID-19 led to a 10.3-per cent increase in unemployment in April 2020. The Current Population Survey showed there were 25 per cent of those employed in April 2019 who did not have a job 12 months later (Cortes and Forsythe 2023). The fallout of losses in employment from coronavirus has been different across work sectors, emphasising established inequities. Those with low pay were worse off, especially as most could not work remotely. Job losses were greater for Hispanic and non-white employees, younger and the less well educated. Black workers fared least well in employment recovery till February 2021. Older workers were retiring more quickly.

In China, Li et al. (2023a) in their study accessed one million users of mobile phones and 71 million records from January 2018 until September 2020. They found unemployment during COVID-19 increased by 72 per cent and claims for government benefits by 57 per cent. Workers over 40 years of age, women and migrants were most affected. Unemployment increased most in hospitality, and in cities relying on exports and healthcare. During natural disasters there are elevated levels of depression and anxiety. During COVID-19 many with job insecurity had poor mental health. Unemployment and labour market transformations were the first consequences of coronavirus. Ibanescu et al. (2023) studied six countries in the EU for job insecurity during the virus and found a clear link, more so in stronger economies.

A report based on two Australian Bureau of Statistics (ABS) surveys conducted in the initial stages of the pandemic (Weekly Payroll Jobs and Wages in Australia, and the Labour Force survey) showed trends were developing around the most disadvantaged workers (Gilfillan 2020). Accommodation and Food services and Arts and Recreation had the greatest rates of job loss.

The most affected of these groups were 20–29-year-olds and 60 years and older. Those aged 40 years and older had the greatest loss of wages. Men were more affected than women in the rate of job loss and in the decline in employment. Full-time workers had a greater employment decline than part-time workers, while casual workers had all aspects of declining employment affected.

Effect on inequity

Labour market inequalities have increased due to mitigating approaches for COVID-19. Work regulation changes have affected different workers in several ways. Inequality intensified. Remote work and other changes have had differential effects. Many essential workers including mobile workers cannot work from home. Edler and Staub (2023) found in Switzerland that having insecure employment was related to increasing labour market flexibility, as was short-term work.

Damar (2023) maintains the pandemic in Turkey 'weakened neoliberalism's' economic system, affecting production, manufacture, capital flow, supply chains and labour. The researcher says the Turkish approach to COVID-19 is based on the principles of neoliberalism including labour market flexibility and deregulation. Similar criticisms were made of the US and Brazil. These approaches to coronavirus governance have been strongly criticised as they put economic indicators and profit before health and lives.

The pandemic had its greatest impact on young people (Ng et al. 2022) Their future career choices have been partially shaped by coronavirus. The co-workers examined the effects of jobs with low pay on the well-being and psychological profile of young people in Singapore. Jobs included delivery, and driving and sales, with most delivery/drivers having no more than a technical certificate. Higher paid workers engaged more in telecommuting and had more work while those with low pay had more disruptions at work and poorer well-being. Higher paid workers were in skilled crafts (such as mechanics), dominated by migrant workers. However, the virus had a greater impact on low paid workers. The low paid young workers need support coming out of the coronavirus. In the pandemic digitisation has led to many administrative jobs at threat of being displaced. In other countries young people have experienced great hardships through COVID-19. Further, Bohlmann, Chitiga-Mabugu and Mushongera (2021) offer an analysis of the structural causes of youth unemployment in South Africa.

ILO (2023c) reports that the growth in global employment in 2023 was expected to be only 1.0 per cent which is about half that of 2022. Unemployment worldwide is expected to rise a little to 5.8 per cent. The size of the increase is due to a tight supply of labour in high-income countries. The slowdown may mean workers have to accept jobs of lesser quality.

COVID-19, globalisation, labour and employment

According to the OECD (2020c) changes that were occurring to labour markets accelerated during the pandemic. Digitisation and automation have increased (note Baldwin 2019a, b; Devaraj et al. 2021). Jobs were created outside high growth areas due to the increase of teleworking. However, there was more pressure in work involving lower education and at risk of automation. Trade opportunities increased due to some reshoring of supply chains. COVID-19 led to work impacts occurring quickly, even though there may only be minor changes in green transition. There are challenges for a reduced and ageing working population. In rural areas, for example, the pandemic will have a greater effect than automation has had.

The pandemic effect for some was devastating. Many people who lost their jobs during the first few months of the pandemic did not return to the labour market quickly. Women were most likely to be first to lose their job and last to re-enter the job market (ILO 2020b). This occurred for many workers with disabilities. These challenges will have a severe effect on efforts to reduce poverty and inequality in the near future, putting achieving Sustainable Development Goals further at risk. They also risk adding discontent and anxiety in the world of work. 'Despite its promises, globalisation – perhaps the most defining feature of the world economy over the last several decades – ... has not always benefited all people and economies. In many countries, income inequality has been rising steeply since the 1980s' (ILO 2020b, 3).

Social exclusion and racial discrimination were common effects of COVID-19 on labour force participation for indigenous people in Australia (Dinku, Hunter and Markham 2020). These reduced their return to gaining much needed work experience. Khama (2020) reported there were millions of migrants in India that anticipated unemployment due to lockdown and potential recession. Many had returned to their villages, and more were waiting for lockdown to end. There was greater risk for those working without written contracts and those nearing the end of their contract.

Heenan and Sturman (2020) use a Marxist perspective in referring to 'socially necessary labour' in an era post-COVID-19 with the world needing to deal with climate change and with a repositioning of labour. Climate change has largely been left out of the debate during COVID-19, even though in Australia where there were devastating bushfires just preceded the epidemic. During COVID-19 some labour was classified as 'essential' before determining socially necessary labour for purposes other than for capital accumulation. COVID-19 has emphasised the fatal weaknesses in delivering access to food, shelter and other basic goods and services using the market. There needs to be a focus in COVID-19 on the relationship between labour and nature. 'An eco socialist perspective ... unites these concerns, and. .... a renewed conversation about the purpose of our collective labour (is needed). In doing so, we can view the COVID-19 and climate crises as different terrains in ongoing class struggle' (Heenan and Sturman 2020, 198). An ecosocialist approach links socialism with a green orientation.

In Australia the government response to COVID-19 has focussed on flexibility and adaptability of state governance and procedures. This has particularly been on employment. There was alternative funding and support for workers and business, especially small business in Australia. This showed that given appropriate circumstances there can be different styles and modes of governance. In a study of businesses, employer organisations, trade unions and government agencies in nine countries their increased inter-relationships provided an effective form of governance in the pandemic (Brandl 2023).

Other effects on the labour market

Several countries are looked at in the effects of the pandemic on labour markets. These include developed economies such as the US, Canada, Italy and Spain and developing economies such as India (as well as China) and in South America. Bogliacino et al. (2023) estimate the effects of labour market shocks on depression, anxiety and stress. These can happen due to poverty, financial crises and recession. Each increased during the pandemic causing the worst outcomes occurring to the most vulnerable groups. Alleviating poverty can have positive effects for mental health. In data from Italy, Spain and the UK the researchers (2023) found these negative mental health outcomes mainly resulted from labour market shock.

Yu et al. (2023) studied the shock from COVID-19 and its effect on industry specialisation and local labour markets in China. The study covered industries in 380 cities from May 2017 to September 2020. The resilient labour market was heterogeneous, affected by industry structure and labour distribution. More diverse labour markets adapted better in the pandemic. Larger cities were most affected. The virus had a significant impact on the internal structure of local job markets. Diversified job markets were more resistant to 'shocks.' The agricultural industry benefitted most through diversification, while finance and information technology (IT) benefitted much less. Yu et al. (2023) recommend that for countries outside China, economic complexity and industrial diversification can help mitigate the effects of future possible pandemics.

Governments have taken radical steps to curb the effects of the virus. Physical distancing has led to some businesses closing and economies being weakened. Protecting the public has had a huge effect on labour markets (Borucka et al. 2023). During the pandemic several countries developed financial measures to support the vulnerable. This included South Korea, Australia, the US and Singapore. COVID-19 had disproportionate effects on household income and on people remaining at work. Non-essential jobs were affected most by physical distancing measures. Low-income self-employed workers were worse off, as well as other self-employed and temporary workers

(Ha 2023). Further, women with childcare responsibilities were also affected by COVID-19 regulations as well as school closures.

Latin America had an economic recession due to COVID-19 (Maurizio et al. 2023). GDP contracted by 6.8 per cent in 2020, The region already had economic slowdown and reversals of labour gains where informal labour and inequality previously existed. Informal workers, those with low skills and women were most affected by the pandemic. The six Latin American countries in the study were Argentina, Brazil, Costa Rica, Mexico, Paraguay and Peru. Informal workers exited the labour force when losing their jobs. Transitions from informal to formal jobs dropped significantly during the virus. Employment rate recovery since mid-2020 has partly been due to an increasing number of informal jobs.

Chatterjee and Dev (2023) maintain that tracking labour market changes is difficult in India due to the size of the population and that significant demographic changes are taking place. Data paucity is a key problem. Using a population-based dataset they report that the effects of COVID-19 are uneven, and recovery depends on the level of education. There were more men than women in full-time jobs.

Agriculture was just one of the industries severely affected by COVID-19, with Eastern Canada an example (Khedhiri 2023). Prior to the virus these markets were healthy: they then became less integrated due to restrictions to travel and labour shortages. In future government needs to develop more resilience in the agricultural industry and less vulnerability to natural shocks.

Losing jobs during COVID-19 happened most in face-to-face contact jobs, and least in essential jobs and remote work (Montenovo et al. 2022). Face-to-face jobs involve the highest risk due to the virus. Some reasons for declining labour supply are compromised childcare arrangements, schooling problems or other family and health requirements. Drawing on the US Current Population Survey, Montenovo et al. (2022) looked at socio-economic factors in labour market responses to coronavirus. Early in the pandemic there was a greater loss of jobs for younger people, Hispanics, and college or high school diploma qualified people. The researchers conclude that gaps in job loss can't be explained by socio-economic differences.

The role of politics

Woods, Schneider and Harknett (2023) claim that there are some polarised beliefs about COVID-19 driven by personalities, especially in the media and politics. The co-workers use the Shift Project (2,039 workers in 89 large companies) to point out that Americans have held deeply divergent views on virus severity, physical distancing and mask wearing. This is partly due to ex-president Donald Trump who 'downplayed' the extent of coronavirus and raised questions over the need for a full government response. Politics had created a lack of compliance by many with interventions to mitigate the virus effect. It also showed the effect of polarisation on work health, especially on the front line. COVID-19 reshaped the labour market, in particular for those working in the service sector, where many had precarious work. Woods et al. (2023) found safety measures at work were related to employees' assessments of personal safety and mental health. However, this was only the case for Biden voters.

Labour market effects across countries

Entrepreneurship influences the labour market. Hean and Chairassamee (2023) studied the effects of COVID-19 and lockdowns on the number of new business applications in the US. There was a variety of business applications, such as those with a high propensity of becoming a business, and ones from a personal service or corporation. During lockdown the number of new business applications reduced significantly. After lockdown, however, the number of applications grew significantly, while applications with a high propensity to becoming a business reduced during lockdown and after.

Füleky and Szapudi (2022) report that states in the US moved in what looked like unison in responding to COVID-19. Labour markets most affected were urban and unemployment was higher in densely populated areas. COVID-19 led to large labour market disruptions in Australia. Initial economic decline related to efforts to combat health effects. There was a significant increase in both unemployment and reduced work hours. Black and Chow (2022) reported that in Australia job mobility declined sharply. People were reluctant to change jobs as JobKeeper (a payment from the government to supplement employer wages) provided stability. The labour market improved significantly in late 2020, and in early 2022 mobility was at its highest in a decade, combined with a strong labour market.

In developed countries work for young people is an important status step to adulthood. COVID-19 has threatened that. Early in 2020 unemployment affected young and to a lesser degree older workers (Li et al. 2023b). In the US's Current Population Survey young adults (20–29 years) between January 2020 and April 2020 had the biggest increase in unemployment, especially for women. In their study of six countries (US, China, Lithuania, Italy Slovenia and Portugal) the researchers (2023b) found that if young people had negative feelings about lockdowns this influenced how their well-being was affected by job/income loss.

Gavriluță, Grecu and Chiriac (2022) discuss the socio-economic framework of the labour market in the EU during coronavirus. The imbalances caused by the virus are based on political decision-making on public health. Social isolation and physical distancing had marked sociopsychological impacts including alienation and anxiety. Having a positive labour market active in employment has beneficial economic effects. Gavriluta et al. (2022) found a deep economic crisis, substantial unemployment and negative growth. This affected women most.

Parwez (2023) engaged with the 'gig' economy. They focussed on precarious work in food delivery that used online platforms during the virus (see Chapter 10, this volume). Customers engage through inexpensive phone and internet connections which enables this form of labour. In 'gig' labour traditional employer/employee relationships are replaced with the workers called 'partners' or contractors. In many cases they have little occupational health and safety (OHS) protection and no sick leave or holiday pay. Employers evade key labour responsibilities. In countries like Australia there have been attempts to regulate the industry. Companies like Uber claim prices will rise if there is industry-wide regulation. Work is highly precarious; incomes are low and there is a danger of accidents if work is in food delivery. Lockdowns during the virus exacerbated problems for these workers.

Migrant and refugee labour

Globally, refugees and migrant workers globally have had poor work and living experiences during COVID-19. Even though engaged in essential jobs many have little safety support and protection from the virus and few work/citizen rights. The situation for many is likely not to improve post-pandemic.

Gheorghiev (2023) addressed economic migrants in the Czech-Republic and their vulnerabilities amid measures to mitigate COVID-19. The researcher looked at the relationship between immigration and labour market composition using a capitalist framework. Migrants from third world nations had access to the country during the pandemic, but they and their families lacked appropriate support and healthcare. This was due to host countries not providing practices, policies and measures of labour market equality.

Due to the Ukrainian invasion over seven million people have left the country, mostly women. In terms of labour market integration women are not a focus of 'integration measures' (Bešić and Aigner 2023). Employment is a key integration issue. Digital literacy was a key issue in social integration for refugees. There was little action from support organisations, so the women relied on families, particularly children for digital learning. There are several problems, however, with refugees' work, including residence permits, legal status, discrimination, health and help with job searching. Coronavirus increased the challenges for refugee women who found themselves without fundamental infrastructure.

Wholesale unemployment, reductions in working hours and pay and negative effects on business and trade resulted from COVID-19. Ndomo, Bontenbal and Lillie (2023) looked at how public health measures affected the labour market position of 17 African migrants with high levels of education in a study (September 2020 to June 2022) in Finland. They were employed in essential jobs in restaurant, transport, healthcare and cleaning. These were typically migrant jobs. They had low status and low skilled employment but job security.

'Migrants have become an increasingly important part of the workforce in many countries in recent years. This is evident in countries that have come to rely more extensively on migrant workers, such as the United Kingdom .... and "nations of immigrants" that have traditionally encouraged permanent settlement, such as Canada and Australia' (Groutsis, Kaabel and Wright 2023). Many migrants have had increasingly precarious work, depending on how they have been defined. In Australia in the 1990s there were social inclusion policies for migrants, but more recently neoliberalist policies have dominated, with economic returns and profitability, and efficient labour organised in employers' interests. This put achieving short-term needs at the cost of humans labouring. Groutsis et al. (2023) refer to this as 'flexible capitalism,' characterised by migrant workers seen as being indifferent and lacking attachment. They are treated as an on-demand commodity. During COVID-19 many countries humanised their migrant programmes and provided these workers with assistance (e.g. UK, Canada, Ireland and Portugal). However, the Australian government made it clear it would not support temporary migrant workers. It called them visitors. While the government introduced JobKeeper (helping businesses and people keep jobs), and JobSeeker (doubling unemployment benefits) there was no support given to migrant labour. Only temporary migrants regarded as in essential work such as food, health, horticulture, hospitality and tourism were tolerated. However, they did not receive welfare support. New Zealanders with temporary visas, however, could access pandemic wage subsidies. Consequently, migrant workers in Australia were dehumanised making for even more precarious conditions during COVID-19.

The pandemic has had a substantial effect on immigrants in the US principally through risk of infection at work. A greater proportion of foreign-born employees than native born worked as frontline essential workers with 70 per cent of immigrants employed this way (Allen, Pacas and Martens 2023). Larger groups of foreign-born employees, especially those who are unauthorised immigrants, have a greater risk of coronavirus exposure than native born employees. Their vulnerability increases due to having no access to health insurance and living in crowded accommodation. Immigrant mortality rates are greater than for native born citizens.

Zhang, Banerjee and Amarshi (2023) describe Canada's immigration policies as changing over three years through COVID-19 and beyond. Migrants will play a key role in national recovery from the virus effects. Express Entry is a hybrid system introduced in 2015, used to admit migrants on a supply/demand basis. The researchers (2023) found this system responsive and flexible and narrows work profiles of incoming migrants. However, employers feel it doesn't address labour gaps fully or gaps in skills. This aspect needs addressing in Express Entry to provide the best mix between migrant labour and employers.

Globally COVID-19 led to substandard working and living conditions of migrant workers. Dutch meat plant working conditions came under particular focus (Berntsen et al. 2023). They had poor employment conditions, employer dependency and poor social connections. With the onset of the pandemic the EU was to guarantee the supply of migrant workers for essential industries. They had little health protection, and their work and rights were scant. Coming after a period of deregulation the state was central to securing migrant workers during the virus. Due to virus outbreaks in Dutch meatworks, there was pressure to improve this precarious work, although this was slow. Berntsen et al. (2023) found that state-related institutional change did not address their work: some organisations became ineffective as protectors of mobile workers, Berntsen and Marino (2023) maintain that worldwide, migrant workers are over-represented in low paid and precarious jobs.

European states pressurised Eastern European governments to allow citizens to travel abroad to be migrant workers. Rumanians travelled to Austria, Germany and the Netherlands to work in fields, and to the UK and other countries for agriculture. Ulceluse and Bender (2022) report these migrant workers were not given protective gear such as masks and hand sanitisers, and physical distancing was not enforced. The researchers (2022) refer to there being a two-tiered system of citizenship in the EU. These workers had de-skilling, abuse, exclusion from services available to the public and an absence of social rights.

Del Real, Crowhurst-Pons and Olave (2023) maintain there was great stress through COVID-19 containment policies by Venezuelan immigrants in Argentina and Chile. These stressors were through loss of income and jobs, having low job status leading to being devalued, and in not being able to send remittances to relatives in need in Venezuela. These factors contributed to anxiety and depression.

Conclusion

The arrival of the COVID-19 pandemic bought with it major changes to the labour market globally. It increased unemployment for a period and exacerbated inequalities in the labour market affecting young people especially, women more than men and people of colour. Effects of the virus were on both developed and developing economies. Most countries had essential services industries where pay and conditions were not always good, and work could not be home-based.

Mobile workers, many of whom were refugees or migrants, had poor conditions for work and living. Even though many migrants and refugees worked at essential jobs they had no access to services such as health, welfare or benefits. There is a need for post-pandemic national and international cooperation to improve these conditions. Also, labour markets need to find a way in the future not to rely on the deregulating effects of neoliberal governance and be prepared for events such as climate change and other pandemics.

12 Gender, COVID-19 and changing globalisation

Recent social movements such as #metoo have focussed on gendered oppression and moved forward the case of equality for women. Further, Beck's risk society is discussed in relation to gendered inequity and is critically evaluated. There is also a discussion on the ways in which globalisation has affected gender relations and the effects of coronavirus disease-19 (COVID-19) and containment measures on gender. Gender-based violence as an outcome of the virus is also presented.

Prior to COVID-19 there were changes to gender relations that saw inroads towards what appeared to be equity in the workplace. In the previous decade social movements had given women in some countries a voice that had long been suppressed. The most public of the social movements was 'Me Too' with Tarana Burke (also #metoo) in the US which started to challenge sexual assault on black women but became a forum for all women to express about gender harassment. The #metoo acted as a voice for all women (Araujo and Peterson 2021). COVID-19 emphasised existing gendered inequities, with women being worse off overall than men. It halted progress in gender equality and exacerbated gender differences, including a gendered division of labour. Unemployment, reduced hours of work and increased domestic labour were more frequent for women during the pandemic.

Women globally have yet to attain parity with men in the labour force. Despite globalisation leading to overcoming many barriers women worldwide do not always get equal pay for equal work, and in developing countries gender inequities persist to a larger degree. Women in developed countries have almost an equal share of the labour market. However, greater inequities were evident during COVID-19 in lockdown where women assumed an unequal role of unpaid home-based labour including childcare and home-based schooling. In addition, during lockdown globally, there was an increase in domestic violence with perpetrators and victims forced to be at home together.

DOI: 10.4324/9781003449423-15

Theoretical issues

Ulrich Beck and his *Risk Society* thesis discusses the role of women in late modernity. He considers individuation and how we see women finding themselves in relation to men, in the family and in the labour force. The extremes of women's experience contain at the least having little or no power and either working for little pay, or not being allowed to work. For women in migrant labour this is often fully supported by government. At the other end of the spectrum is the woman who can, within limits, choose her destiny. Yet women are constrained by laws and customs which limit their opportunities for free choice.

Skelton (2005) investigated tension and struggles in academia (men and women and between women in different strata). She explored the use of Beck's concept of the individualised individual in terms of understanding actions and attitudes of people in modern society. Beck's theory of individualisation looks at western societies as no longer being first modernity, having moved to a second, reflexive modernity. They are in transition. Beck referred to the 1970s when change and social movements started. According to the researcher (2005) three factors in shaping the second modernity occurred: the breaking down of class divisions (note Beck and Beck-Gernsheim 2002); women started becoming liberated from gender roles; and the nature of work changed. These led to the 'individualized individual' – people at the centre of action (Beck 1992). Skelton (2005, 320) claims a major flaw in Beck's concept relates to his theory that '"power" is a finite resource operating at macro levels which thus fails to embrace understandings of "power" that allow for micro-political struggles.' In first modernity Beck sees women as powerless in relation to men but fails to outline power imbalances between women occupying different positions in a hierarchy. For Beck's individualised individual model to be more useful in interpreting the position of women in the second modernity, a more nuanced discussion of power is needed. Further, feminists need to recognise and engage with tensions and power struggles between women in academia.

Mulinari and Sandell (2009) point out that Beck (1992) and Giddens (1991, 1992) refer to the processes of individualisation and reflexivity. This is where people shape their own biographies. These processes lead to changes in gender and family relations. Women are individualised in the modern family. Beck refers to it leading to a crisis in gender and family relations, one that must be resolved. He sees the labour market threatening the family: the state should intervene in this conflict (e.g. by providing childcare). Mulinari and Sandell (2009) respond that it is women individualising that brings about changes in the family. They also query Beck's position on reproductive work. If women are individualised who will do that work? The researchers (2009) refer to women's role in late modernity as being employed on an equal footing with men, and in a family but not necessarily engaged in reproduction.

Globalisation and gender

Neoliberal globalisation has flourished during the last few decades. The free market approach with free trade and deregulated labour markets have benefitted some, as shown by the amazing wealth some individuals have accumulated. Others have contributed to this wealth by providing cheap sources of labour in a globalised world. In one of these groups, women who serve as mobile workers for wealthier countries, have little or no work safety protection and few if any citizen rights. They work mostly under state orchestrated mobile arrangements.

In some developed countries populist governments have enjoyed increasing success. Migration and conservative views on sex and gender have played a part in their popularity. In 2016 Brexit occurred, where the UK left the EU, with an anti-migrant vote and conservative values coming to the fore. The Black Lives Matter movement occurred a little later. Donald Trump became President of the US espousing conservative attitudes about women which some considered sexist. A large issue in conservative parts of America is opposition to the right to an abortion.

The rise of populist right-wing parties is a result of cultural backlash, a reaction to social liberalist values. The conservatives have attracted an anti-gender movement against equality and lesbian, gay, bisexual, transgender, intersex, queer/questioning, asexual (LGBTQI +) rights. Off (2023) maintains that the cultural backlash includes socio-economic factors, anti-immigration issues and gender. Sweden is a very gender equal country. Before coronavirus there had been the 'Women's Marches;' and the #metoo movement. In Sweden a contentious consent law had been passed. With gender issues important the Swedish Democrats, a populist right-wing party, became the third largest party. As identified by post-election data, voters with more conservative gender issues followed by anti-immigration beliefs voted for the populist party.

There has been increasing female participation in the labour market in middle and higher-income countries. This has left a gap in domestic labour and care, regarded as women's work. There has been labour migration to the global South. The gap is being filled by women from poorer countries. There are many levels involved in the moving of these women's bodies, including households, industries and governments and a belief these women can migrate out of poverty. Malaysia is one destination for migrant labour while Indonesia and the Philippines are suppliers. Spitzer et al. (2023) collected multifaceted and interview data of migrant domestic workers from a variety of agencies. Domestic labourers in Malaysia have no labour laws protecting them. While satisfied with healthcare access they experienced long-term separation from their families, poor pay and little control over their work, resulting in stress. They used self-sacrifice as a way of explaining their situation which is based on structural inequalities. This refers to a situation of palliative coping where they are powerless to act. Neoliberal policy incorporates marketisation, privatisation and commercialisation and has led to all three countries (Indonesia, the Philippines and Malaysia) benefitting at the cost of the well-being of these migrant workers.

Globalisation and gender have been examined in the context of international relations, borders, trade, welfare and migration (Ullah et al. 2023). Traditionally, power held by men has been seen as decentralised, thus aiding women. Counter to this view is that globalisation reproduces gender stereotypes. Those favouring globalisation's positive effect on women support the view that employment opportunities for women are gained in 'export processing' (companies allowed to import goods and then export without duty) and companies relocating have given women more professional mobility. Southeast Asia is an example of this. However, the pandemic has shown that women carry the heaviest weight of domestic responsibilities, including childcare. Certain feminists argue that women's labour is more expendable and cheaper and that multinational organisations tend to support patriarchal systems.

Globalisation has enhanced economic growth in some developing countries. Economic growth has supported some gender equality. Farooq et al. (2020) report on globalisation and gender parity in the 47 member countries of the Organisation of Islamic Cooperation (OIC) between 1991 and 2017. A negative aspect of globalisation on the economy has occurred in most of those countries, and there was a positive impact on high-income countries only. Moves towards gender equality in the workforce aided economies.

Robertson, Lopez-Acevedo and Savchenko (2020) studied gender and pay differences in Cambodia and Sri Lanka where women participate less in the labour market than men. However, freeing up trade, especially in apparel, has created opportunities for women in these countries, moving mainly from agriculture. Women working in the export sector are vulnerable to falling prices. They benefit in terms of better pay in the apparel industry, but their pay and conditions depend on the global market. Robertson et al. (2020) maintain in Morocco globalisation has disrupted life as is the case for many women in the Global South, and affected children left at home when women migrate in search of jobs. When migrating, both women and men have few rights. In addition, global capitalism assumes women are suited only for low paying jobs.

Private investment, tourism and exports are at the base of Morocco's economy. The relocation of businesses to Morocco has meant it, and its labour market has become more dependent on the world economy. Fajardo Fernández, Soriano-Miras and Trinidad Requena (2023) argue that leaving a parent's home means less division of tasks by gender. In the family home task allocation was made by the father and the mother carried out the household routine. If leaving home single women should only move into same sex accommodation. Women have a low occupational status in industries that have been relocated and may seek other options, such as marriage. However, ascending the organisational hierarchy may mean having to adopt a masculine-like role.

Asongu and Odhiambo (2023) argue there are four aspects of economic inclusion in sub-Saharan Africa. These are that women are very much under-represented in economic sectors: more women being involved would improve the human face of the sector; a greater inclusion would allow some United Nations (UN) goals to be met; and their inclusion would fill some important gaps in the scientific literature. The lack of representation of women is much more evident in political and economic spheres in the sub-Sahara African region. Most women work in agriculture and petty trading. Asongu and Odhiambo (2023) based their study on 35 countries in the region from 1995 to 2019. Political and economic globalisation have positive influences on women's employment in agriculture and is driven by globalised trade. Social globalisation has negative effects on women's agricultural employment, affected by the impact of information and culture. Globalisation has a negative effect on women's involvement in industry, but positively affects women's employment in service organisations.

The gender pay gap has gained a lot of public and academic attention. Using the European Working Conditions Survey Antón et al. (2023) studied a ten-year period of gender pay differences in the EU. They found the position of women deteriorated in environment and quality, and there was a catch-up process in non-monetary aspects of work.

Gender responses to COVID-19

There were gender differences in responses to COVID-19. Men died more frequently than women and had more serious symptoms. Yet once severe symptoms were experienced the death rate for women and men were similar.

Being older and having a greater number of comorbidities were related to mortality and disease severity for both SARS and COVID-19 (Jin et al. 2020). Men's cases were more serious. Men died at 2.4 times the rate as women of coronavirus. Prevalence was equal between the genders, but men faced worse outcomes. Mukherjee and Pahan (2021) argue that these occurrences may be a result of differences in ACE2 receptor and TMPRSS2 (serene protease). They may be attributed to sex differences in the immune response. Differential gender responses could also be due to factors such as comorbidities and smoking. In a review Gebhard et al. (2020) found that men in China had a fatality rate from COVID-19 of 2.8 per cent, compared to 1.7 per cent for women. European data show aged men had more severe consequences.

With SARS-CoV-1 infection in 2003 women had a lower risk of death. With SARS-CoV-2 women also had a lower mortality risk suggesting there is a sex-dependent susceptibility in both cases: women have better resistance overall to viral infections. Raimondi et al. (2021) studied 431 patients in Italy with COVID-19 and found women were about one-third of the male population in hospitals. In addition, severity of disease and 28-day mortality was less frequent for women. Risk of dying while having the disease is not affected by gender. In less developed countries women and men may have different opportunities in accessing health services. Raimondi et al. (2021) found that women hospitalised with the virus were less likely than men to die. However, when severe disease is present, risk of dying is similar for both women and men.

Labour process and gender

Layoffs and challenges in combining work and home care, as well as childcare and domestic labour, have affected women most. Lockdowns were particularly difficult times. Aslam and Adams (2022) refer to stay-at-home mothers being forgotten during the pandemic. Their home was always their workplace. Whereas in dual income households there may have been some inroads for males taking more domestic responsibilities. In single income households there is less impetus to change. Aslam and Adams (2022) used a Marxist-feminist analysis of domestic labour for women and a labour process approach focussing on skill, autonomy and resistance. In their qualitative study they found that control and autonomy for home-based women deteriorated during lockdown, thus affecting the labour process. Amid school closures they had to focus on child-based activities. Although partners were spending more time at home, this disrupted the women's work rhythm, and criticisms aimed at them enflamed the situation. This led to 'mom guilt' and feelings of inadequacy, often leading them to set impossible standards for themselves, based on a neoliberal logic around individual responsibility. The emphasis on partners' paid employment together with increased childcare requirements and less autonomy increased gender differences at home. Based on labour process analysis and an understanding of 'motherwork' the home can be seen as a gendered work environment and altered domestic labour can exacerbate gender inequities hidden at home.

Gender and COVID-19

Some regard COVID-19 to be an outcome of neoliberal globalization with open markets, trade and borders, creating an environment where a virus could spread, unabated. Public health measures and state interventions meant a series of measures including physical distancing, isolating and lockdowns were implemented. As these measures meant people became home-based women more than men had poor outcomes: this included more home-related responsibilities, more childcare and more home schooling. Also, the rates of domestic violence during lockdown increased. Compared to men, a greater proportion of women became unemployed or had their hours of work reduced.

In developed countries, while having an equal representation in the labour force, women do a disproportionate amount of housework. Alon et al. (2020) report the gap in gender pay is, for women, 'like childbirth.' However disproportionate gendered outcomes also relate to expectations and norms.

There were globally 1.5 billion children not in school in the early stages of the pandemic. Many families looked after children themselves, most likely affecting mothers more. In the pandemic women had most negative effects on their employment opportunities. Closures of childcare centres had a major effect on working mothers. 'Many businesses are now becoming much more aware of the childcare needs of their employees and respond by rapidly adopting more flexible work schedules and telecommuting options. Through learning by doing and changing norms, some of these changes are likely to prove persistent' (Alon et al. 2020, 2). Flexible working arrangements are likely to exist post-pandemic, and this will help to promote gender equality. In addition, more males are taking on childcare, and this may reform the norms about household division of labour.

Madgavkar et al. (2020) report that globally job loss for women during coronavirus was 1.8 times higher than for men. Women around the world account for 39 per cent of employment, but 54 per cent of job losses. They also have an unequal burden of unpaid care. In South Asia, North Africa and the Middle East, women's share of unpaid work is between 80 and 90 per cent. Women's jobs were more at risk than men's during the pandemic. COVID-19 highlighted how training and education identifying gender roles and stereotypes and perception of risk can help to underline the roots of inequality. Acting on gender inequity now could improve the lives of millions of women and add substantially to economic growth across the world.

Flor et al. (2022) maintain that during the pandemic sex and gendered health and well-being have not been well studied. They examined data from 193 countries. Gender differences in social, health and economic spheres have been found. The indirect effects of COVID-19 for women are disadvantage and marginalisation. These include increased vaccine hesitancy, reproductive services disruptions and an upsurge of violence against women at home. Females were more likely to drop out of school. However, the researchers (2022) report they found there were no gender differences in vaccine hesitancy, although this has been questioned by some writers. The most significant gaps are in the workforce and unpaid labour. The smallest gender gaps have been found in the wealthier countries, and the largest gaps in Latin America, sub-Saharan Africa and the Caribbean.

Nivakoski et al. (2022) report there were gender differences in paid and unpaid work during coronavirus. COVID-19 emphasised existing inequities in gender, with men being better off than women overall. The pandemic stopped progress in equalising gender as well as the division of labour.

According to Bonaccorsi et al. (2023) almost 60 per cent of the world population use the Internet and 55 per cent of Europeans had searched for health information on the Internet and more so in Denmark and Germany. While there is good, accurate information there is also a lot of disinformation, especially during the pandemic. Those using least online health information have been older, male, of low socio-economic status and low education. The researchers et al. (2023) investigated gender differences amongst Italian university students. While male students had higher scores on digital health literacy (DHL), female students sought more information for themselves and others about coronavirus, and other topics. '(F)emale students have proven to have a lower DHL, to be less satisfied with the information, to use different research sources and to consider very important different facets of information. On the other hand, males seem to adopt more heuristic behaviours' (Bonaccorsi et al. 2023, 10).

Vaccination

In Europe women were found to be significantly less likely to state an intention to be vaccinated against the virus than men, a finding different to that Flor et al. (2022) reported previously. Vaccine hesitancy was greater amongst women as was refusal to be vaccinated (Toshkov 2023). Yet women were more likely to see COVID-19 as a serious health issue. In the study of 27 European countries, conflicts were found over which gender was against vaccination (other than for coronavirus) in general. Women showed more trust in medical information from sources such as social networks and the Internet. However, they had less trust in health authorities and had a lower perceived risk of infection. One explanation of this vaccine hesitancy is their belief vaccines are ineffective and unsafe, with risks being greater than benefits.

Vaccine hesitancy is a problem in controlling COVID-19. The following groups have been associated with it: young people, females, those on low incomes, with a low education, having a low trust in medicine and from smaller ethnic groups. In addition, there are those who don't see themselves having a risk from the virus, and those who use particular social media sites, as well as those subscribing to conspiracy theories. Allington et al. (2023) conducted an online survey of adults in the UK in late 2020. They found high reliance on information from social media, not being reliant on print or broadcasting sources, being of white ethnic origin, and having low trust in scientists and government affected vaccine hesitancy. However, there was little evidence to explain age and gender causes. The study suggests that vaccine hesitancy is also strongly tied to both conspiracy suspicions and attitudes to vaccines in general. This presents a unique challenge for public health organisations and government vaccination programmes, which need to combat misinformation to ensure COVID-19 vaccination.

Other gendered factors

Elomäki and Kantola (2023) investigated the European Parliament's response to COVID-19 by looking at how effective the feminist governance framework was in gendered aspects. Previous research on COVID-19 has focussed on the visibility of women making decisions during crises, the gendered effects of the virus and ways to make these gender receptive. The researchers (2023) use feminist governance to look at mechanisms to forward gender equity during the virus. In political organisations this can either enable gender perspectives or it can reduce frameworks for gender equality. In times of crisis feminist governance may be put aside. It refers to a dedicated gender equity component and gender mainstreaming (involving an integrated gender perspective). Feminist governance was successful in the European Parliament in bringing in a gender perspective to the pandemic. The Parliament had previously not adopted a gendered approach to the 2008 Global Financial Crisis.

Gender equality is a UN sustainable development goal. However, Caldarulo et al. (2022) confirm that women do more unpaid work than men, work in unequally gendered workplaces and have more responsibility for unpaid work at home. During COVID-19 their unpaid work increased, including caring for children and elderly relatives, and doing home schooling. Working mothers were 5 per cent more likely to reduce working hours than working fathers and 7 per cent more likely to change how they worked. In terms of professions science, engineering and technology as well as mathematics see women disproportionately under-represented. These areas are based on existing hierarchical structures. Progress on redressing the balance has been hindered by COVID-19 measures to contain the virus. Investigations showed that virus measures contributed to gender disparities in universities and other workplaces (universities studied were from R1 Carnegie research organisations). Women had increased childcare responsibilities and domestic labour. There were significant impacts on reducing research activities, and work and life balance of women.

Businesses employing mainly female and part-time workers on low pay were most affected by COVID-19 (Singh, Shirazi and Turetken 2022). Gender pay inequity increased during COVID-19 and was more evident in the private sphere, due to a stronger presence of collective bargaining and unions in the public sphere. This Canadian study confirmed gender gaps in employment and the lower pay for women.

Carreras, Vera and Visconti (2023) investigated gender differences in relation to public health measures for COVID-19 in Peru. There was a disproportionate effect of lockdown on women's lives as was the case in many developing countries. Women were likely to be exposed to sexual harassment and domestic violence and have a greater share of domestic responsibilities. The co-workers found that women supported lockdown measures more than men and complied more with recommendations about avoiding crowds and gatherings in public.

Gender-based violence

Family violence was a problem during lockdowns where household members were confined to home for extended periods of time. Substantial fines were set for those individuals who did not comply with lockdowns.

Family and victim professionals have cited that physical distancing and stay-at-home orders during COVID-19 had increased the rate of family violence. According to Drotning et al. (2023, 189) 'family violence as verbal abuse, physical abuse, or restriction of access to a cell phone or the internet, (is) perpetrated by a member of the household against another member of the household.' In the US in April 2020 family violence was 15 per cent higher than the year before. In Australia, China and Spain 'intimate partner violence' was higher during than before the pandemic. In Spain there was a 23 per cent increase in women reporting this violence during a three-month lockdown early in the pandemic.

Gender-based violence has been labelled by the UN as a 'shadow epidemic' (Aborisade 2022). This has been the case in Nigeria for example. A relevant theoretical approach to explaining sexual violence during lockdown in Nigeria is crime opportunity theory. This is based on selecting targets who provide high rewards for little effort. It also draws on routine activity theory which argues a suitable target is needed, the offender is motivated, and there is no effective guardian available. African research into COVID-19 has largely not addressed gender violence. The researcher (2022) reported on this qualitative study of 19 girls and women who had experienced gender violence during coronavirus lockdown, including incest, marital rape and date rape. Lockdown increased vulnerability and provided opportunities for the offenders.

Zulver, Cookson and Fuentes (2021) also discuss the shadow epidemic of gender violence which swelled during lockdown, this time in South America. Cosas de Muieres, a WhatsApp digital platform was developed in response to gender-based violence in the event of mass migration to and through Columbia from Venezuelia. The apps' function was to give information about services available in case of gendered violence and to collect data to inform for more effective gender-based programmes. A Gender Data Kit has been developed and this applies a feminist perspective from data collected. The researchers (2021) found that early in the pandemic problems were emerging globally and that feminists had a role to play in documenting unintended outcome of public health policies. Even when presenting policy and decision-makers with gender-based violence data, there needs to be the political will to deal with it. Those who work with the Cosas de Muieres programme have a responsibility to the women who contribute data to it that health policies are presented, and decision-makers are confronted with the findings.

Domestic and gender-based violence is gaining in importance over recent decades. Home confinement approaches for COVID-19 have created a worse situation. The pandemic had already led to increased anxiety, depression and stress. That stress had already been exacerbated by employment and economic problems for families (Rodriguez-Jimenez, Fares-Otero and García-Fernández 2023). In Spain, forced confinement in the home occurred with perpetrators and victims being together. Data based on Spain's helpline on calls requesting advice and help for domestic violence show that between April and June 2020 there was an increase in calls compared to the previous two years. This increase started to decline after lockdown finished in July. By September calls to the helpline decreased to the pre-pandemic levels of two years previously.

Related gender effects of COVID-19

A study of whether the gender of CEOs during COVID-19 affected investors' behaviour was carried out in South Korea. Shin and Park (2023) examined publicly listed businesses in Korea and found abnormal returns '(30, 60 and 90 days)' were less negative for companies where the CEO was a woman. This provides some evidence that for investors, in times of acute crisis female CEO's leadership is preferred.

The experience of 1.5 million Italian students in mathematics and reading were examined for effects of the pandemic. They had primary/lower secondary education in 2020–21 and were compared with a pre-COVID-19 cohort from 2018 to 2019 (Borgonovi and Ferrara 2023). The COVID-19 group had experienced school closures, lockdowns and other disruptions to their lives and education. Previous middle-level achieving students were affected most by the virus. The gender gap for secondary school students was the least. This was also the case in reading only for those in primary school. Low achieving primary school boys had an achievement gap in reading compared to 2018–19. The researchers (2023) suggest that the virus and mitigation strategies may have disrupted teacher and peer stereotypes on mathematics for girls and reading for the boys, thereby reducing the gender gap for all.

Fake news appears to be news, is misleading and is deliberate. There has been a large increase in fake news with COVID-19, and it is most evident on social media where there are billions of users worldwide. It is a public health risk. There are no fact checks or control over posts. Many people believe the following fake news: the virus is transmitted by mosquitoes, that epidemics can be cured by pure alcohol and that coronavirus is a biochemical weapon. Wu and Mustafa (2023) carried out an online survey of 300 social media users in China. Previous studies have shown males are less susceptible to fake news, but the co-workers found this not to be the case. A larger sample is needed.

Conclusion

Gender issues related to the pandemic have shown that in a crisis women may bear an unequal load. Globalisation has made us aware of the disadvantages that many women around the globe experience. Decision-makers at the local level need to provide support to women who in many cases are working in lower paid jobs and managing high levels of domestic labour.

At the level of the state, policy needs enacting in equality for women both in the labour market and in the context of home/family responsibilities. Globally there are benefits from having more and better employment of women.

Policymakers in planning for future crises need to consider that women may have been more affected by COVID-19. They need to look at providing extra resources for women to equalise their experience.

13 Labour process and socio-political contexts

A view to the future

A sociological perspective is helpful in considering economic and political contexts of globalisation. This includes Beck's *Risk Society* thesis and the resurgence of other sociological approaches including that by Bryan Turner. In Chapter 13, a labour process approach is summarised, analysed and discussed in relation to a changing social, occupational and economic landscape resulting from coronavirus disease-19 (COVID-19). There is also an analysis of advances in technology that have occurred as a result of coronavirus. A political economy perspective helps to explain the economic, social and political perspectives in relation to the response to COVID-19, and of the measures used to mitigate the virus. The last part of the chapter deals with the theme of how we can apply what we have learned from the COVID-19 experience to other global threats such as future pandemics and global warming/climate change.

Beck's (2000a) position on globalisation was evaluated in Chapter 2 (this volume). Sociologists such as Turner (2010b) evaluate globalisation, prior to COVID-19. Other sociological studies contribute to understanding the effects of coronavirus. Lupton (2020) presents three sociological theories and how they help in understanding digitisation during coronavirus in Chapter 7. In Chapter 11 Beck (1992) is discussed in relation to COVID-19 and labour markets, and in Chapter 12 in arguments on gender.

COVID-19 has been a global bad (note Beck 1992). Mythen (2005) is critical of risk society theorists such as Beck because they ignore how political discourse can reinforce hegemonic interests. The change from industrial modernity to risk society entailed a basic move in political economy. This represented a shift from producing social goods (such as health and wealth) to the production of social bads (such as pollution). She (2005) claims that the political economy has not had a fundamental shift: social distribution has not been reconfigured by risk. Social bads such as COVID-19 affect the rich and poor alike, but the poor and vulnerable were most exposed to the virus and in many cases have no health or medical cover. Alaszewski (2021) further evaluates Beck's *Risk Society*. Giddens (1991) and others provide explanations relevant to COVID-19. Gavrila and Cilento (2022) look at Beck and global risk in relation to the pandemic and the war in Ukraine.

DOI: 10.4324/9781003449423-16

Mythen (2021) argues that Beck's *Risk Society* thesis presents threat over time and that the unpredictable quality of risk has potentially apocalyptic consequences for the world. Beck distinguished between natural hazards caused by external agents. In industrial society medicine, science and technology can control natural hazards. From the late 1970s, environmental risk makes society confront the effects of capitalist development – this includes global warming/climate change. Criticism of the risk society thesis centres around its generality and its lack of sensitivity to differences in geography, culture and history.

In Beck's *Risk Society* he refers to producing and distributing risks in the second modernity. Society's structure is based on risk. Hazards result from risk such as diseases occurring from globalisation, for example COVID-19. Managed by scientists they can affect anyone. The speed of the spread of the virus shows the vulnerability of societies today. In his analysis, while saying class is less important Beck states that risks may bring inequalities (Constantinou 2021).

The media plays a significant role in the perception of risk. Wang and Mao (2021) studied the role of Chinese newspapers in reporting the pandemic. They looked at Beck's interpretation of media. According to Beck (2009) there is a time when media causes harm through a collective silence, thereby maintaining the current social order. In the initial stages of risk, there is a belief that scientists can control risk (note Beck 1992). At other times media can turn risks into catastrophes, where there are not sufficient resources to control the situation. Using treatment responsibility and consequences, coronavirus changed from being a risk to catastrophe. Chinese journalists moved from playing down the virus to presenting it as a national catastrophe then to reporting it as a global crisis.

COVID-19 and the labour process

This includes lessons learned about national and international governance. Research using labour process theory has looked at the effects of the work from home edict as a response to coronavirus.

COVID-19 had a significant impact on agriculture and its trade. Coronavirus outbreaks in the global North and indirect impacts of lockdown measures on the global South have been important. Morton (2020) uses a framework previously used with the HIV/AIDS pandemic to examine the impact of COVID-19 on agriculture in developing countries. This refers to susceptibility to infection, resistance to infection, vulnerability of households and communities and resilience to the impact of the virus. He (2020) looked at aspects of labour process that make people more susceptible. In developing agricultural value chains different technologies, space and reliance on businesses are gained. It also shows differing relationships of power between purchasers and sellers, employers and workers and between government and other agencies. Field labourers are engaged in physically distanced activities, while those in packing venues and in processing are likely to be more vulnerable to infection. This includes those in purchasing and selling in traditional markets.

Labour process entails production including tools, the design of jobs and worker management relations incorporating power differences and social relations. Labour process theory examines relations at work under capitalism. As a result of COVID-19 some employees were required to work from home and felt some increased control due to this. Home-based work enhances worker agency. But there is a caution. Digital technologies control these workers as part of the labour process (Bromfield 2022). Another working at home problem is extending time spent on work, which may be less controlled than in the office workspace. Also the lack of face-to-face interaction with colleagues can be problematic although there are digital alternatives. It can represent disrupted social relations of production.

Technology, the labour process and COVID-19

The pandemic has drawn a global response to protect nations as well as economic responses. These include increasing welfare to deal with the economic fallout. It has driven digitisation and technology to the forefront at a far greater rate of uptake and development than before the pandemic. The changes to digitisation, use of metrics and general technological advances have been at unprecedented levels. They have had implications for the way work is carried out, much of which has been home based. They have also led to increased surveillance as a result of the home lives of many workers.

Technology has an impact on the labour process and also on responses to coronavirus. According to Hodder (2020) surveillance, control and resistance have been the focus on the effects of technology on work and this helps in understanding the effects of COVID-19 on work. Changes to the labour process over time (as many employees have been 'estranged' from workplaces) should be seen in relation to new technology. Surveillance and control of frontline coronavirus workers, and of those working from home was a key interest of the labour process for Hodder (2020). This changed the contours of control. Before COVID-19 electronic monitoring and work intensification were already problematic for emergency workers and those working from home. For home-based workers, electronic monitoring can lead to losing leisure. This new work intensification has become the new normal. Employees work as if they are permanently online and more subject to management control. Zoom, Teams, mobile phones and more have become part of the work arsenal, blurring home/work boundaries. There has been resistance to these new technologies. Unions in many countries have lost ground but are an important source of resistance to unregulated technological change. Facebook and other social platforms have been used for work. In the UK unions and collective action by workers have reported on inadequate protection from coronavirus. In this sense technology is socially mediated (Hodder 2020).

The provision of information services and products continued through COVID-19 when labour intensive (and/or physical producers) shut down or drastically reduced operations. Information technology has played a key role where needed. As a result of the pandemic organisations have strived to digitise services and products, including online banking and digital payments (Seetharaman 2020). Coronavirus has meant organisations sought digital solutions for products and services to provide safety by minimising physical contact. The development of new ecosystem organisations requires resilience and adaptability to an increased rate of change.

Political economy of COVID-19

There are many uncertainties in the period moving forward from COVID-19. For example, there may be other pandemics waiting to happen and there are issues of global warming/climate change. Owing to the degree of mobilisation to control and contain COVID-19 the world may have a better understanding of how to respond better in dealing with future pandemics, climate change and other threats.

Political economy and socio-political approaches apply to COVID-19. Used by Adam Smith, the term political economy referred to how government policies influence life in the real world. Owing to the degree of mobilisation to control and contain COVID-19 the world should be more able to deal with crises in the future (Peterson and Walker 2022). There are relevant sociological theories that account for both political and social influences. An understanding of socio-political factors and of political economy is essential for addressing the future. Milfont, Osborne and Sibley (2022) maintain there was an increase in socio-political efficacy with successful lockdowns in New Zealand. This efficacy increased pro-environmental outlooks, including beliefs about climate change.

Virus effects on colonial lines

With COVID-19, 'morbidity and mortality are far worse for indigenous people, migrants, black people, and other victims of racism, discrimination, and marginalisation' (Bump et al. 2021, 1). This is based on differences in educational opportunity and access to care and wealth. Physical distancing opportunities were also less for these groups. People employed who were most affected were in low paid jobs and many in essential work. Poor people suffered more than the rich, and international competition is likely to have harmed the global South most due to a lack of vaccines and medicines. According to Bump et al. (2021) these latter countries have the least political and economic bargaining power. The political economy of coronavirus relates to the effects of the virus, how affected countries act and consequent power relations. It is based on extraction, consequent of long-term modes of exploitation established in a colonial period, opposing the principle of public health and working towards a global solution to the pandemic. This process is the opposite to United Nations principles. 'These processes of colonialism and extraction and their effects explain much about the inequitable political economy of COVID-19 and point to some possible remedies' (Bump et al. 2021, 1).

The slow response to the pandemic in the US laid bare the 'structural inequalities' of racism, creating a recipe for structural vulnerability for this pandemic (Bailey and Moon 2020). By early May 2020, the US recorded over 30 per cent of global cases for infection and over 28 per cent of the world's death toll (given under-reporting in some less developed countries). The Bronx was used as a case study undertaken of structural inequalities where divesting systems were based in racism and devaluing 'black and brown' lives. Several pejorative terms were used for the virus by the government in the initial stages. These included a 'Democratic hoax' and the 'Chinese flu.'

Virus response by government

Political and economic systems affected the impact and spread of coronavirus (Karabulut et al. 2021). A question is what is the degree to which liberal democracies protect their populations? Using five indicators of democracy this study showed that while the infection rates of the virus appear to be higher in more democratised countries, they have lower case fatality rates. The relationship between case fatality rate and censorship of media by government is negative but is positive in relation to rate of infection. The co-workers say other styles of government act faster to mobilise their citizens. While populations may follow instructions carefully they often lack transparency and have overly stringent responses. Censoring information about the pandemic may make people less cautious: controlling media may create vulnerability. Corruption may lead to serious response problems as does unequal access to resources. Regarding lower death rates in liberal democracies, it may be because they have more developed and accessible health systems.

In terms of considering the political economy of hysteria, mass and digital media connected with government had negative consequences during COVID-19 (Bagus, Peña-Ramos and Sánchez-Bayón 2021). If there are no state restrictions, mass hysteria might result. In the pandemic if role models die it may lead to hysteria. Negative effects depend on the size of the state.

Questions have been raised about the draconian isolation policies for the virus in India. Kaplan, Lefler and Zilberman (2022) suggest that political and economic issues may have been the motivation for these policies. This was especially the case for developing countries, where there was such a high social and economic cost to the pandemic, and investment in research and development, vaccines and monitoring technologies is required. Generally, the cost of COVID-19 was a result of under preparation and underinvestment, particularly in mitigation approaches and prevention, which could be a lesson for the future.

Neoliberal effects

Some have said that coronavirus is the end of neoliberalism. Paulsson and Koglin (2023) report that in Sweden passenger numbers on public transport significantly decreased as a result of COVID-19, initially by 20 per cent. There was a decision to reduce the number of services but unions and others opposed this. The services resumed but income from ticket sales dropped markedly. The researchers (2023) report that the drivers tried to save the situation to avoid a collapse. The effect of the pandemic on marketisation of the transport system put it under severe stress. Paulsson and Koglin (2023) question whether actions of the operators represent a move from neoliberal policies. The rules of marketisation were unchanged, but the actions regarding marketisation were to protect neoliberal policies.

COVID-19 shone a light on the drawbacks of having homes treated as financial investments. These emerged as part of the political economy in neoliberal Canada. August (2021) discusses a new type of housing ownership managed by large capital rich entities in Canada. Returns are maximised to investors. Financialisation of seniors' and multifamily housing began more than a decade ago. At that time there were government cuts to funding which paved the way for private investment. Finance operators own 33 per cent of all seniors' housing companies. Solutions would include moving to 'definancialised sectors' and socialised ownership. States could make a priority of having secure and affordable housing, rather than for profit. During coronavirus death rates were highest in financialised owned accommodation, creating a crisis. This showed shortcomings of private sector ownership. Since COVID-19 in Australia and other countries a focus has been on providing affordable housing and rentals, given high inflation levels. The government is investing in social housing, and this is to try and create some housing equality.

Effects on unions

Trade unions have been facing challenges and reduced membership, particularly when confronted with COVID-19. Hunt and Connolly (2023) studied the impact on trade unions of COVID-19. Interviews of union officials mainly in the UK were conducted during the second wave of coronavirus, seven months since the start of the pandemic. The study found that unions were making accelerated changes to how they operate under the new circumstances and this includes adapting to new technologies. Activism and engagement of members had increased including online activity and most unions had adopted new ways of recruiting, communicating, campaigning, representing and negotiating. Confidence within unions is important for their renewal.

Politics

During COVID-19 32 per cent of all destinations around the world closed their borders in February 2021. Virus containment measures such as stay-at-home rulings bought domestic tourism to a halt (Okafor and Yan 2022). Death rates from coronavirus negatively impacted on tourism recovery as did physical distancing policies. Also, most people preferred not to take part in leisure that involved crowds. There was no correlation between vaccination rates and tourism recovery. Lee (2022) investigated the extent to which lockdown measures for COVID-19 were due to state governors' election issues in the US, and the amount of attention there was to death reduction and economic loss. Political concerns rather than virus issues were the main focus. Governors with elections forthcoming instituted longer lockdowns that were more stringent.

A political economy perspective of the COVID-19 crisis can be employed to see how private and public bodies are responding and renegotiating. One aspect of this is the disruption of forms of governance, over and above public health and economic crises. These disruptions have implications beyond the pandemic (Cotula 2021).

Preparation for future pandemics and climate change

Bickley et al. (2021) argue that there needs to be more research with COVID-19 on whether global disease forecasting using the 'globalization index' and considering social, political and economic elements should be undertaken to aid future planning for pandemics and climate change. The prediction of time delays in the emergence and transmission of disease through nations' borders would help in forecasting in the future. The virus had a great effect on political economy. Relations are based on power differences, and issues of governance at state and global level. The pandemic has drawn a global response in protecting nations and economic responses including increasing welfare to deal with the economic fallout. Lessons learned about national and international governance are paramount. An underlying theme of the book is how can we apply what we have learned from the COVID-19 experience to other global threats in the future. Owing to the extent of mobilisation to control and contain COVID-19 the world may deal better with future shocks. It has drawn a global response in protecting nations. It has driven digitisation and technology to the forefront at a far greater rate of uptake and development than before the COVID-19 pandemic. These have had implications for performing work. It has led to increased surveillance as a result on the home lives of many workers. This may overshadow gains in work and home balance for many employees.

Those who trust in science believed in mobilising against COVID-19. A belief in science has fuelled the response to COVID-19: could this belief translate into addressing climate change? However, many don't trust or believe in climate science (see Chapter 9, this volume). Both COVID-19 and climate change 'share the same microeconomic foundations, involving an overprovision of a global public bad. In addition, they entail externalities whose correction comes at very high economic and social costs' (Fuentes et al. 2020). There is no evidence that climate change hastens the spread of COVID-19, but there is evidence that in regions with poor quality air people with coronavirus are more likely to die. These issues are important in estimating how climate change needs to factor in supportive governance.

Humanitarian crises

Zarocostas (2023) reports in the *Lancet* that currently there is a major global humanitarian crisis. Factors contributing are the deteriorating climate crisis, armed conflict, epidemics and economic slowdown. This affects 339 million people in 68 countries and is a 25-per cent increase from the start of 2022. Countries include DRC (Congo), Afghanistan, Nigeria, Ethiopia, Ukraine, South Sudan, Somalia, Syria and Yemen. Israel and Gaza in late 2023 were also affected. The crisis is affected by COVID-19, Ebola virus disease, vector-borne diseases and cholera. Climate change is steadily increasing vulnerability and risk. Those countries contributing least to climate change are greatest at risk. COVID-19 and war have caused a need to reconsider humanitarian ecosystems, and capacity building with aid is needed with health information, human resources and supply chains.

Sustainability

Hodder (2020) maintains that rethinking the future of work after COVID-19 will shift the focus to skills, the value of work and inequality. The pace and types of governance shifts, as well as the range of alliances and interests, and the ways of countervailing power, might change from long established patterns. These need investigating. Further, how might the pandemic crisis cause instability in political circles with the more recent upsurge in populist parties (Cotula 2021)?

In Australia, automation and the development of robots is not advanced, and there has been a lack of innovation and skills and training investment which has undermined competitiveness (Dean et al. 2021). Government needs to create conducive social and economic conditions broadly. COVID-19 has emphasised the need to be self-sufficient in manufacturing and to rely less on weak global supply chains. Australia has a natural supply of resources for renewable energy. Carbon-based sources of energy are reducing in importance and fossil fuel prices are increasing. Energy transitions need to meet the requirements of climate change. Australia is equipped for economic reconstruction post-pandemic. The researchers (2021) refer to work on the labour process, economic geography and political economy to look at the impact of the Fourth Industrial Revolutions and how it might affect the Australian economy. Its future lies in renewable energy.

COVID-19 has increased the need to combine social environment, sustainability and economic goals into the management of supply chains as well as coordinating business practices. Khurana et al. (2021) argue that instead of the neoliberal emphasis on profitability the goals of enterprises should be to contribute to people and the planet's future. The upheavals of the pandemic should lead to making companies COVID-19 resilient. There needs to be balance between human, economic and ecological goals. Wholesale improvements can emerge out of adversities. The pressures from stakeholders and investors can lead the way in sustainable developments. Economic development is more important than economic growth in coming out of the pandemic. Khurana et al. (2021) sought to identify the factors important to making India more resilient to the effects of the virus, to climate change and other future shocks. Survival of future companies depends on their sustainability and resilient supply chains. Manufacture is expected to move from China to India. The future in global events lies in creating sustainable manufacture supply chains, socially, ecologically and with resilience. Governance was *the* most crucial factor involved in the rebuilding of societies and industries and helping them become more resilient with future shocks.

COVID-19 was managed reasonably in Africa creating useful pathways for managing climate change (Ongoma et al. 2023). In the pandemic top political governance and innovations met coronavirus challenges as well as leadership from the African Centers for Disease Control and Prevention. Resources including data were successfully shared to limit the virus. Africa is least well prepared to deal with the effects of climate change. Coordinated international mitigation and adaptation is needed to reduce the growing risks. Internationalism and the governance of networks that dealt well with COVID-19 should form African approaches to climate change. These can work through practical-oriented leadership providing leverage in confronting environmental issues.

Impact of neoliberal globalisation

Coronavirus has demonstrated a need to change for the future. In most cases governments have agreed to change but this has not occurred. Universal Health Coverage (UHC) has not happened in all countries and this impeded responses to the pandemic as many people were excluded from medical and healthcare. In future this kind of care that can only come from public funding may protect from pandemics occurring or slow their passage. UHC needs to include all marginalised groups and in culturally appropriate ways. Due to the impact of neoliberal globalisation socio-political systems need to become more resilient by addressing inequities. In order to deal with global warming/

climate change there needs to be reform of governance. The form of governance that was successful in protecting against infections and death can help to address the crisis in climate change. In addition, regulating the relations between multinational corporations and governments could come a long way to providing fairer and more equitable governance.

Some reasons for the transmission of the virus were globalised trade and the mobility of people. According to Bickley et al. (2021) more globally connected countries and particularly cities are associated with disease transmission. However, globalised countries were less likely to adopt protective policies for COVID-19. Those countries with greater political globalisation may be more willing to learn from others. Globalisation increases growth, and any restrictions to combat the virus (such as with travel) are likely to come at a cost. Travel restrictions appeared to be one of the major factors in slowing the spread of the virus. The researchers (2021) report that while more globalised nations applied international travel restrictions earlier, they did so when their virus case numbers were higher. Also, countries tended to implement policies similar to their economic partner(s), rather than to neighbouring countries.

Garel and Petit-Romec (2021) argue that financial issues due to COVID-19 have created uncertainties over future climate action. Companies that are responsible about environment had better stock returns during the pandemic: that is in reducing energy consumption and emissions. Those with a longer-term perspective did best. Investors rewarded climate orientation more, as a result of the virus. This is encouraging for the future as much that occurs in the corporate and business environment is shaped by investments.

From the virus – A possible way forward

Fuentes et al. (2020) compared COVID-19 and global warming/climate change to see how the pandemic can inform climate change mitigation. 'The COVID-19 crisis is itself a reality check for climate policy, international governance and prevention in general; the COVID-19 pandemic is a mock laboratory of climate change, where the time scale of unfolding events is reduced from decades to days' (Fuentes et al. 2020, 1). Both crises have similar structures, similar economic issues and policy responses. COVID-19 responses may provide insights to policies for climate change. A change of attitudes and behaviour orchestrated by new social norms is possible, including our residential location and leisure activities. These can influence trends in carbon emissions. In a post-coronavirus world, it may be that there will be some emphasis on low physical contact, although this does not seem to be the case more than three years after the pandemic was declared. With coronavirus changes occurred daily, while climate change occurs over the long term.

Economic cost is one reason that organisations, industries and governments have not engaged with measures to combat climate change. With COVID-19 the UK, Mexico and Spain experienced extremely high economic costs. Increasing carbon prices is seen as an overwhelming burden to some. 'This suggests a need for a much deeper social change coupled with a green transformation that decouples economic activity and carbon emissions' (Fuentes et al. 2020, 9). The cost of inactivity is incomprehensible. Sustainable advocates say the costs of solutions to problems of climate change have been overstated. Changes in behaviour underscoring climate change can be accomplished as they were in COVID-19 (with its combination of mandated and voluntary measures such as mask wearing and maintaining a physical distance for the virus).

Both COVID-19 and climate change have needed global action collectively (Meijers et al. 2022). The pandemic had quickly adopted behavioural change largely not shown with climate change. Using an online survey the co-workers looked at drivers of behavioural change for both global threats. These included threats, both personal and to significant others, fear, participation extent, 'social norms' and perception of government policy. Three drivers for acting on climate change were a changing view of government policy, the threat to significant others and beliefs in the efficacy of participation.

Kirby (2022) writing in the *Lancet* discussed the work of Marion Koopmans who helped launch the Pandemic and Disaster Preparedness Centre initiated by the Erasmus Medical Center in Rotterdam, the Netherlands. She wants global readiness for the next pandemic. The Center focusses on infectious disease, but also how climate change intersects which causes rises in sea levels, complex social and ecological threats and extreme weather. These can bring future health events and disease outbreaks.

The pandemic has affected the well-being of numerous young people and children physically and psychologically (Sormunen et al. 2022). They argue that health promoting schools are essential to deal with effects of the pandemic and prepare school communities for challenges such as climate change. School closures led to learning loss and widened the gap in inequity. Schools provide a unique opportunity to contribute to the well-being and health for young people as well as teachers. Youth and children's literacy is needed with global concerns starting with making sense of COVID-19 and its impact and including under nutrition, obesity and climate change. It calls for attention to washing hands and making a healthy lifestyle, understanding inequities exposed through the pandemic and helping to make school an environment that promotes universal health. Many students had a ragged experience of school. School connectedness is also important for including teachers and non-teaching staff. A bottom-up and democratic approach is needed for participating in intervention programmes targeting the effects of coronavirus and of future crises. For health promotion in schools, empowering and collaborative activities teaching relevant skills and values reflecting a comprehensive approach is needed.

Meeting climate change goals is the most urgent global dilemma. The timing and scope are comprehensive. All social aspects are affected

(Bulder et al. 2022). Resources in top down policies used for coronavirus may work for climate change governance, and a focus on inclusion and solidarity may lead to a more inclusive governance. Some say disruptions caused by the virus will not affect climate change governance. Others say international cooperation is declining due to nationalistic and populist movements. According to the researchers (2022) the governance of climate change is diverse using market or network approaches and is hierarchical. In looking at the imposition of lockdowns, these happened by top down means, showing that this approach can work in an emergency. The process of greater government intervention flies in the face of neoliberalism which has eroded the welfare state and left states and communities at the whims of the market. The same applies to climate change. In dealing with climate change, behaviour would need to change where people could see their actions having meaningful effects on reducing emissions.

Bulder et al. (2022) report a hierarchical approach to dealing with climate change, and for government to set regulations while communicating effectively. A 'composite hybrid' approach is required. The commercial sector needs subsidies, investment, research and taxation incentives to help with energy transition. The co-workers add that some market-based governance is needed. Bottom-up and participatory action as well as governance of networks are required together with improved data management between government and community bodies. COVID-19 will have a long-term influence on governments and governance used in crises. There is a need for large-scale public investment and a regulatory role of government.

Conclusion

The key issue emerging from the book is what are the lessons we have learned from the virus that can help in preparing for future crises? The role of sociopolitical factors in understanding the pandemic is important. It provides the context for how COVID-19 was managed and for those who endured most effects. Together with a labour process approach they are important tools of sociological analysis. The neoliberal approach may have hastened the spread of COVID-19 and government increased its role in the pandemic including returning in some cases to elements of welfare to protect states. Styles of governance recommended include hybrid approaches. Using the open market as the driver simply won't work as the base. A problem has been that a lot of activity has happened at the local level, but this cannot progress without commitment at the level of national/state government and international level. Lessons learned from COVID-19 testify to a greater role of government while incorporating changes and influences from the 'grass roots' level.

References

Abeysinghe, S., V. Amir, N. Huda, F. Humam, A. F. Lokopessy, P. V. Sari, et al. 2022. "Risk and Responsibility: Lay Perceptions of COVID-19 Risk and the 'Ignorant Imagined Other' in Indonesia." *Health, Risk and Society* 24 (5–6): 187–207. https://doi.org/10.1080/13698575.2022.2091751.

Abidi, N., M. El Herradi, and S. Sakha. 2022. "Digitalization and resilience: Firm-level evidence during the COVID-19 pandemic." *IMF Working Papers*. No. 2022/034 International Monetary Fund. https://www.imf.org/en/Publications/WP/Issues/2022/02/18/Digitalization-and-Resilience-Firm-level-Evidence-During-the-COVID-19-Pandemic-513169 (accessed August 29, 2023).

Aborisade, R. A. 2022. "COVID-19 and Gender-Based Violence: Investigating the 'Shadow Pandemic' of Sexual Violence during Crisis Lockdown in Nigeria." *International Journal of Offender Therapy and Comparative Criminology*. https://doi.org/10.1177/0306624X221102781.

Adair, T. 2022. "How Has COVID-19 Impacted Australia's Life Expectancy." *Nossal Institute for Global Health*. University of Melbourne. https://mspgh.unimelb.edu.au/centres-institutes/nossal-institute-for-global-health/news-and-events/how-has-covid-19-impacted-australias-life-expectancy#:~:text=Analysis%20of%20the%20latest%20available,three%2Dquarters%20of%20these%20declines (accessed August 31, 2023)

Adekola, J., D. Fischbacher-Smith, T. Okey-Adibe, and J. Audu. 2022. "Strategies to Build Trust and COVID-19 Vaccine Confidence and Engagement among Minority Groups in Scotland." *International Journal of Disaster Risk Science* 13 (6), 890–902. https://doi.org/10.1007/s13753-022-00458-7.

Ahmad, M., and E. Satrovic. 2023. "How Do Transportation-Based Environmental Taxation and Globalization Contribute to Ecological Sustainability?" *Ecological Informatics* 74. 102009. https://doi.org/10.1016/j.ecoinf.2023.102009.

Ahmed, I., M. Ahmad, J. J. P. C. Rodrigues, G. Jeon, and S. Din. 2021. "A Deep Learning-Based Social Distance Monitoring Framework for COVID-19." *Sustainable Cities and Society* 65. 102571–102571. https://doi.org/10.1016/j.scs.2020.102571.

AKIXI. 2021. "The long and short-term effects of COVID-19 on employee wellbeing." *AKIXI.* https://www.akixi.com/news-and-events/impact-of-covid-19-on-employee-wellbeing/ (accessed September 2, 2023).

Alaszewski, A. 2021. "Plus ça Change? The COVID-19 Pandemic as Continuity and Change as Reflected Through Risk Theory." *Health, Risk and Society* 23 (7–8): 289–303. https://doi.org/10.1080/13698575.2021.2016656.

Albert, M. 2023. "Climate Emergency and Securitization Politics: Towards a Climate Politics of the Extraordinary." *Globalizations* 20 (4): 533–547. https://doi.org/10.1080/14747731.2022.2117501.

AlBloushi, A. F. 2022. "Contribution of Saudi Arabia to Regional and Global Publications on COVID-19–Related Research: A Bibliometric and Visualization Analysis." *Journal of Infection and Public Health* 15 (7): 709–719. https://doi.org/10.1016/j.jiph.2022.05.013.

Alcalde, A., and J. E. Escribano 2020. "Will COVID-19 end globalisation?" *Pursuit*. University of Melbourne, May 2020. https://pursuit.unimelb.edu.au/articles/will-covid-19-end-globalisation (accessed August 20, 2023).

Allen, R., J. D. Pacas, and Z. Martens. 2023. "Immigrant Legal Status among Essential Frontline Workers in the United States during the COVID-19 Pandemic Era." *The International Migration Review* 57 (2): 521–556. https://doi.org/10.1177/01979183221127277.

Allington, D., S. McAndrew, V. Moxham-Hall, and B. Duffy. 2023. "Coronavirus Conspiracy Suspicions, General Vaccine Attitudes, Trust and Coronavirus Information Source as Predictors of Vaccine Hesitancy among UK Residents during the COVID-19 Pandemic." *Psychological Medicine* 53 (1): 236–247. https://doi.org/10.1017/S0033291721001434.

Al-Maroof, R. S., S. A. Salloum, A. E. Hassanien, and K. Shaalan. 2020." Fear from COVID-19 and Technology Adoption: The Impact of Google Meet during Coronavirus Pandemic." *Interactive Learning Environments*. https://doi.org/10.1080/10494820.2020.1830121.

Alon, T., M. Drepke, J. Olmstead-Rumsey, and M. Tertilt. 2020. "The impact of COVID-19 on gender equality." *National Bureau of Economic Research*. NBER Working Paper 26947. https://www.nber.org/system/files/working_papers/w26947/w26947.pdf (accessed September 3, 2022).

Alon, T., M. Kim, D. Lagakos, and M. Van Vuren. 2023. "Macroeconomic Effects of COVID-19 across the World Income Distribution." *IMF Economic Review* 71 (1): 99–147. https://doi.org/10.1057/s41308-022-00182-8.

Altman, S. A. 2020. "Will COVID-19 have a lasting impact on globalisation?" *Harvard Business Review*. May. https://hbr.org/2020/05/will-covid-19-have-a-lasting-impact-on-globalization (accessed September 10, 2023).

Altman, S. A., and C. R. Bastian. 2022. "The state of globalisation in 2022." *Harvard Business Review*. April. https://hbr.org/2022/04/the-state-of-globalization-in-2022 (accessed September 1, 2023).

Ancillo, A de L., T. del Val, and S. G. Gavrila. 2021. "Workplace Change within the COVID-19 Context: A Grounded Theory Approach." *Economic Research-Ekonomska Istraživanja* 34: (1): 2297–2316. https://doi.org/10.1080/1331677X.2020.1862689.

Anderson, J., L. Rainie, and E. A. Vogels. 2021. "Experts Say the 'new Normal' in 2025 Will Be Far More Tech-Driven, Presenting More Big Challenges." Pew Research Centre. https://www.pewresearch.org/internet/2021/02/18/experts-say-the-new-normal-in-2025-will-be-far-more-tech-driven-presenting-more-big-challenges/ (accessed August 22, 2022).

Angheluţă, P. S, and C. G. V. Badea. 2018. "The Green Economy Influence on the Urban Sustainable Development." *Economics, Management, and Financial Markets* 13 (3): 315–326.

Antipova, A. 2021. "Analysis of the COVID-19 Impacts on Employment and Unemployment across the Multi-Dimensional Social Disadvantaged Areas." *Social Sciences and Humanities Open* 4 (1). https://doi.org/10.1016/j.ssaho.2021.100224.

Antón, J.-I., R. Grande, R. Muñoz de Bustillo and F. Pinto. 2023. "Gender Gaps in Working Conditions." *Social Indicators Research* 166 (1): 53–83. https://doi.org/10.1007/s11205-022-03035-z.

Araujo, N., and C. L. Peterson. 2021. "The 'Me Too' Movement, Gender and Risk." In *Identifying and Managing Risk at Work: Emerging Issues in the Context of Globalisation*. Edited by C. L. Peterson, 173–187. Abingdon: Routledge. https://doi.org/10.4324/9781315223339-12.

Asada-Miyakawa, C. 2021. "Pandemic impact highlights need for resilient Occupational Safety and Health systems." International Labour Organisation (ILO). https://www.ilo.org/asia/media-centre/news/WCMS_782022/lang--en/index.htm (accessed August 21, 2023).

Asayama, S. 2015. "Catastrophism Toward 'Opening Up' or 'Closing Down? Going Beyond the Apocalyptic Future and Geoengineering." *Current Sociology* 63 (1): 89–93. https://doi.org/10.1177/0011392114559849.

Aslam, A., and T. L. Adams. 2022. ""The Workload Is Staggering": Changing Working Conditions of Stay-at-Home Mothers Under COVID-19 Lockdowns." *Gender, Work, and Organization* 29 (6): 1764–1778. https://doi.org/10.1111/gwao.12870.

Asongu, S. A., and N. M. Odhiambo. 2023. "Economic Sectors and Globalization Channels to Gender Economic Inclusion in Sub-Saharan Africa." *Women's Studies International Forum* 98: 102729. https://doi.org/10.1016/j.wsif.2023.102729.

Assefa, Y., C. F. Gilks, S. Reid, R. van de Pas, D. G. Gete, and W. Van Damme. 2022. "Analysis of the COVID-19 Pandemic: Lessons towards a More Effective Response to Public Health Emergencies." *Global Health* 18 10. https://doi.org/10.1186/s12992-022-00805-9.

Attwell, K. 2023. "Project to Explore Impact of Vaccine Mandates." University of Western Australia. https://www.uwa.edu.au/news/Article/2023/March/Project-to-explore-impact-of-COVID-vaccine-mandates (accessed September 1, 2023).

Aubin, D., C. Riche, V. Vande Water, and I. La Jeunesse. 2019. "The Adaptive Capacity of Local Water Basin Authorities to Climate Change: The Thau Lagoon Basin in France." *The Science of the Total Environment* 651 (Pt 2): 2013–2023. https://doi.org/10.1016/j.scitotenv.2018.10.078.

August, M. 2021. "Financialization of Housing from Cradle to Grave: COVID-19, Seniors' Housing, and Multifamily Rental Housing in Canada." *Studies in Political Economy* 102 (3): 289–308. https://doi.org/10.1080/07078552.2021.2000207.

Axon, S., A. Bertan, M. Graziano, E. Cross, A. Smith, K. Axon, et al. 2023. "The US Blue New Deal: What Does It Mean for Just Transitions, Sustainability, and Resilience of the Blue Economy?" *The Geographical Journal* 189 (2): 271–282. https://doi.org/10.1111/geoj.12434.

Ayres, J. M. 2004. "Framing Collective Action against Neoliberalism: The Case of the Anti-Globalization Movement." *Journal of World-Systems Research* 10 (1): 11–34. https://doi.org/10.5195/jwsr.2004.311.

Bærenholdt, J. O., and J. W. Meged. 2023. "Navigating Urban Tourism Planning in a Late-Pandemic World: The Copenhagen Case." *Cities* 136. https://doi.org/10.1016/j.cities.2023.104236.

Bagus, P., J. A. Peña-Ramos, and A. Sánchez-Bayón. 2021. "COVID-19 and the Political Economy of Mass Hysteria." *International Journal of Environmental Research and Public Health* 18 (4): 1376. https://doi.org/10.3390/ijerph18041376.

Bailey, Z. D., and J. R. Moon. 2020. "Racism and the Political Economy of COVID-19: Will We Continue to Resurrect the Past?" *Journal of Health Politics, Policy and Law* 45 (6): 937–950. https://doi.org/10.1215/03616878-8641481.

Baird, J., R. Plummer, and O. Bodin. 2016. "Collaborative Governance for Climate Change Adaptation in Canada: Experimenting with Adaptive Co-Management." *Regional Environmental Change* 16 (3): 747–758. https://doi.org/10.1007/s10113-015-0790-5.

Baldwin, R. 2019a. "Globalisation, automation and the history of work: Looking back to understand the future." *VOX: CEPR.* https://unctad.org/news/globalisation-automation-and-history-work-looking-back-understand-future (accessed August 25, 2022).

Baldwin, R. 2019b. *The Globotics Upheaval: Globalisation, Robotics and the Future of Work.* New York: Oxford University Press.

Bankova, Y., and H. Kutsarov. 2022. "Strategies and Tactics for OHS Management to Confront the Pandemic Crisis in the Hospitality Industry: The Case of Countries in Europe." In *Handbook of Research on Key Dimensions of Occupational Safety and Health Protection Management.* Edited by Z. Snežana, B. Krstić, and T. Rađenović, 261–283. Hershey: IGI Global. https://doi.org/10.4018/978-1-7998-8189-6.ch013.

Barak, N., U. Sommer, and N. Mualam 2021. "Urban Attributes and the Spread of COVID-19: The Effects of Density, Compliance and Socio-Political Factors in Israel." *The Science of the Total Environment* 793: 148626–148626. https://doi.org/10.1016/j.scitotenv.2021.148626.

Bardsley, D. K., and A. Knierim. 2020. "Hegel, Beck and the Reconceptualization of Ecological Risk: The Example of Australian Agriculture." *Journal of Rural Studies* 80: 503–512. https://doi.org/10.1016/j.jrurstud.2020.10.034.

Barnett, P., and P. Bagshaw. 2020. "Neoliberalism: What It Is, How It Affects Health and What to Do About It." *New Zealand Medical Journal* 133 (1512): 76–84.

Baru, R. V., and M. Mohan. 2018. "Globalisation and Neoliberalism as Structural Drivers of Health Inequities." *Health Research Policy and Systems* 16: 91. https://doi.org/10.1186/s12961-018-0365-2,

Basu, S. 2023. "Three Decades of Social Construction of Technology: Dynamic Yet Fuzzy? The Methodological Conundrum." *Social Epistemology* 37 (3): 259–275. https://doi.org/10.1080/02691728.2022.2120783.

Bauer, L., K. Broady, W. Edelberg, and J. O'Donnell. 2020. "Ten facts about COVID-19 and the US economy." The Brookings Institute. https://www.brookings.edu/research/ten-facts-about-covid-19-and-the-u-s-economy/ (accessed September 1, 2022).

BBC. 2020. "Coronavirus: How the world of work may change forever." *BBC Worklife.* https://www.bbc.com/worklife/article/20201023-coronavirus-how-will-the-pandemic-change-the-way-we-work (accessed September 1, 2022).

Beaverstock, J. V., R. Cohen, A. Rogers, and S. Vertovec. 2023. "Covid-19 and Global Networks: Reframing Our Understanding of Globalization and Transnationalism." *Global Networks (Oxford)* 23 (1): 9–13. https://doi.org/10.1111/glob.12425.

Becchio, G., and G. Leghissa. 2016. *The Origins of Neoliberalism: Insights from Economics and Philosophy.* Abingdon: Routledge. https://doi.org/10.4324/9781315849263.

Beck, U. 1992. *Risk Society: Towards a New Modernity*. London: Sage.

Beck, U. 1999. *World Risk Society*. Cambridge: Polity Press.

Beck, U. 2000a. *What Is Globalisation?* Cambridge: Polity Press.

Beck, U. 2000b. "Risk Society Revisited: Theory, Politics, and Research Programs." In *The Risk Society and Beyond: Critical Issues for Social Theory*. Edited by B. Y. Adam, U. Beck, and J. van Loon, 211–229. London: Sage. https://doi.org/10.4135/9781446219539.

Beck, U. 2006a. "Living in the World Risk Society." *Economy and Society* 35 (3): 329–345.

Beck, U. 2006b. *Cosmopolitan Vision*. Cambridge: Polity Press.

Beck, U. 2009. "Critical Theory of World Risk Society: A Cosmopolitan Vision." *Constellations* 16 (1): 3–22. https://doi.org/10.1111/j.1467-8675.2009.00534.x.

Beck, U. 2010. "Climate for Change, or How to Create a Green Modernity?" *Theory, Culture and Society* 27 (2–3): 254–266. https://doi.org/10.1177/0263276409358729.

Beck, U. 2011. "We Do Not Live in an Age of Cosmopolitanism but in an Age of Cosmopolitinization: The Global Other in Our Midst." *Irish Journal of Sociology* 19 (1): 16–34. https://doi.org/10.7227/IJS.19.1.2.

Beck, U. 2015. "Emancipatory Catastrophism: What Does It Mean to Climate Change and Risk Society?" *Current Sociology* 63 (1): 75–88. https://doi.org/10.1177/0011392114559951.

Beck, U. 2016. *The Metamorphosis of the World: How Climate Change Is Transforming Our Concept of the World*. Boston: Polity Press. https://doi.org/10.1086/692904.

Beck, U., and E. Beck-Gernsheim. 2002. *Individualisation*. London: Sage. https://doi.org/10.4135/9781446218693.

Beck, U., and E. Beck-Gernsheim. 2009. "Global Generations and the Trap of Methodological Nationalism for a Cosmopolitan Turn in the Sociology of Youth and Generation." *European Sociological Review* 25 (1): 25–36. https://doi.org/10.1093/esr/jcn032.

Beck, U., A. Giddens, and S. Lash. 1994. *Reflexive Modernization Politics, Tradition and Aesthetics in the Modern Social Order*. Stanford: Stanford University Press.

Beck, U., and G. Grande. 2012. "Cosmopolitanism and Cosmopolitanization." In *Blackwell Encyclopedias in Social Sciences: The Wiley-Blackwell Encyclopedia of Globalization*. Vol 1, 306–309. Chichester: Wiley-Blackwell. https://doi.org/10.1002/9780470670590.wbeog113.

Becker, J. C., L. Hartwich, and S. A. Haslan. 2021. "Neoliberalism Can Reduce Well-Being by Promoting a Sense of Social Disconnection, Competition, and Loneliness." *Social Psychology*. https://doi.org/10.1111/bjso.12438.

Beland, L.-P., A. Broder, and T. Wright. 2020. "The short-term economic consequences of COVID-19: Exposure to disease, remote work and government response." Discussion paper 13159. *A Z A. Institute of Labour Economics*. https://www.econstor.eu/bitstream/10419/216471/1/dp13159.pdf (accessed August 24, 2022).

Berntsen, L., A. Böcker, T. De Lange, S. Mantu, and N. Skowronek. 2023. "State of Care for EU Mobile Workers' Rights in the Dutch Meat Sector in Times of, and Beyond, COVID-19." *International Journal of Sociology and Social Policy* 43 (3/4): 356–369. https://doi.org/10.1108/IJSSP-06-2022-0163.

Berntsen, L., and S. Marino. 2023. "Guest Editorial: State Policies and Regulations towards Migrant Work in Times of, and Beyond, the COVID-19 Pandemic." *International Journal of Sociology and Social Policy* 43 (3/4): 293–305. https://doi.org/10.1108/IJSSP-04-2023-547.

Bertilsson, M. 1990. "The Role of Science and Technology in a Risk Society: Comments and Reflections on Beck." *Industrial Crisis Quarterly* 4 (2): 141–148. https://doi.org/10.1177/108602669000400204.

Bešić, A., and P. Aigner. 2023. "Action, Reaction and Resignation: How Refugee Women and Support Organisations Respond to Labour Market Integration Challenges during the Covid-19 Pandemic." *Journal of International Management* 29 (3): 101031. https://doi.org/10.1016/j.intman.2023.101031.

Bianchi, F., G. Bianchi, and D. Song. 2021. "The Long-Term Impact of the COVID-19 Unemployment Shock on Life Expectancy and Mortality Rates." *National Bureau of Economic Research*. Working paper 28304. https://doi.org/10.3386/w28304.

Bicchieri, C., E. Fatas, A. Aldama, A. Casas, I. Deshpande, M. Lauro, et al. 2021. "In Science We (Should) Trust: Expectations and Compliance across Nine Countries during the COVID-19 Pandemic." *PLoS ONE* 16 (6): e0252892. https://doi.org/10.1371/journal.pone.0252892.

Bickley, S. J., H. F. Chan, A. Skali, D. Stadelmann, and B. Torgler. 2021. "How Does Globalization Affect COVID-19 Responses?" *Global Health* 17 57. https://doi.org/10.1186/s12992-021-00677-5.

Black, S., and E. Chow. 2022. "Job mobility in Australia during the COVID-19 pandemic." Reserve Bank of Australia. *Bulletin*, Australian Economy. June 2022. rba.gov.au/publications/bulletin/2022/jun/job-mobility-in-australia-during-the-covid-19-pandemic.html (accessed September 1, 2022).

Boehm, S., and C. Schumer. 2023. "10 Big Findings from the IPCC Report on Climate Change." World Resources Institute. https://www.wri.org/insights/2023-ipcc-ar6-synthesis-report-climate-change-findings (accessed September 1, 2023).

Bogliacino, F. F., C. C. Codagnone, F. F. Folkvord, and F. F. Lupiáñez-Villanueva. 2023. "The Impact of Labour Market Shocks on Mental Health: Evidence from the Covid-19 First Wave." *Economia Politica (Bologna, Italy)* 1–32. https://doi.org/10.1007/s40888-023-00304-z.

Bohlmann, J. A., M. Chitiga-Mabugu and D. Mushongera. 2021. "Youth and Unemployment: Our Present Problem and a Missed Opportunity." *Africa Today* 68 (2): 142–148. https://doi.org/10.2979/africatoday.68.2.07.

Bonaccorsi, G., V. Gallinoro, A. Guida, C. Morittu, V. Ferro Allodola, V. Lastrucci, et al. 2023. "Digital Health Literacy and Information-Seeking in the Era of COVID-19: Gender Differences Emerged from a Florentine University Experience." *International Journal of Environmental Research and Public Health* 20 (3): 2611.https://doi.org/10.3390/ijerph20032611.

Borgen Project. 2018. "The top 10 most important current global issues." https://borgenproject.org/top-10-current-global-issues/ (accessed August 31, 2022).

Borgonovi, F., and A. Ferrara. 2023. "COVID-19 and Inequalities in Educational Achievement in Italy." *Research in Social Stratification and Mobility* 83: 100760–100760. https://doi.org/10.1016/j.rssm.2023.100760.

Bort, S., and A. Kieser. 2023. "Coping with Devils and Climate Change with the Help of Asceticism? Exploring the Role of Asceticism as Trigger of Collective Climate Action." *Environmental Values*. https://doi.org/10.3197/0963271 23X16702350862764.

Borucka, A., M. Chapska, E. Żaboklicka, and R. Parczewski. 2023. "Assessment of the Labour Market during the COVID-19 Pandemic." *Polish Political Science* 52 (1): 149–164. https://doi.org/10.15804/ppsy202236.

Bowen, A., K. Kuralbayvea, and E. L. Lipoe. 2018. "Characterising Green Employment: The Impacts of 'Greening' on Workforce Composition." *Energy Economics* 72: 263–275. https://doi.org/10.1016/j.eneco.2018.03.015.

Brandl, B. 2023. "The Cooperation between Business Organizations, Trade Unions, and the State during the COVID-19 Pandemic: A Comparative Analysis of the Nature of the Tripartite Relationship." *Industrial Relations (Berkeley)* 62 (2): 145–171. https://doi.org/10.1111/irel.12300.

Brennetot, A. 2015. "The Geographical and Ethical Origins of Neoliberalism: The Walter Lippmann Colloquium and the Foundations of a New Geopolitical Order." *Political Geography* 49: 30–39. https://doi.org/10.1016/j.polgeo.2015.06.007.

Briggs, E. A. J., D. Lloyd, and L. Telford. 2020. "New Hope or Old Futures in Disguise? Neoliberalism, the Covid-19 Pandemic and the Possibility for Social Change." *International Journal of Sociology and Social Policy*. https://doi.org/10.1108/IJSSP-07-2020-0268.

Briken, K., S. Chillas, M. Krzywdzinski, and A. Marks. 2017."Labour Process Theory and The New Digital Workplace." In *The New Digital Workplace: How New Technologies Revolutionise Work* Edited by K. Briken, S. Chillas, M. Krzywdzinski, and A. Marks, 1–17. London: Palgrave Macmillan.

Brink, E., and C. Wamsler. 2018. "Collaborative Governance for Climate Change Adaptation: Mapping Citizen–Municipality Interactions." *Environmental Policy and Governance* 28 (2): 82–97. https://doi.org/10.1002/eet.1795.

Bromfield, S. M. 2022. "Worker Agency Versus Wellbeing in the Enforced Work-From-Home Arrangement during COVID-19: A Labour Process Analysis." *Challenges* 13 (1): 11. https://doi.org/10.3390/challe13010011.

Brown, D., M.-C. Brisbois, M. Lacey-Barnacle, T. Foxon, C. Copeland, and G. Mininni. 2023. "The Green New Deal: Historical Insights and Local Prospects in the United Kingdom (UK)." *Ecological Economics* 205: 107696. https://doi.org/10.1016/j.ecolecon.2022.107696.

Budd, J., B. S. Miller, E. M. Manning, V. Lampos, M. Zhuang, M. Edelstein, et al. 2020. "Digital Technologies in the Public-Health Response to COVID-19." *Nature Medicine* 26: 1183–1192. https://doi.org/10.1038/s41591-020-1011-4.

Budimir, S., T. Probst, and C. Pieh. 2021. "Coping Strategies and Mental Health during COVID-19 Lockdown." *Journal of Mental Health (Abingdon, England)* 30 (2): 156–163. https://doi.org/10.1080/09638237.2021.1875412.

Budzi, J. 2022. "Crisis of Neoliberalism and the COVID-19 Pandemic: Reclaiming the Welfare State." *African Journal of Development Studies* 12 (1): 49–69. https://doi.org/10.31920/2634-3649/2022/v12n1a3.

Bulder, C., I. Todd, D. McCauley, and M. K. Burns. 2022. "The Influence of COVID-19 on Modes of Governance for Climate Change—Expert Views from the Netherlands and the UK." *Environmental Policy and Governance.* 1–13. https://doi.org/10.1002/eet.2042.

Bump, J. B., F. Baum, M. Sakornsin, R. Yates, and K. Hofman. 2021. "Political Economy of COVID-19: Extractive, Regressive, Competitive." *BMJ* 372 (73). https://doi.org/10.1136/bmj.n73.

Burgess, A., J. Wardman, and G. Mythen. 2018. "Considering Risk: Placing the Work of Ulrich Beck in Context." *Journal of Risk Research* 21 (1): 1–5. https://doi.org/10.1080/13669877.2017.1383075.

Burns, T. R., and N. Machado. 2010. "Technology, Complexity, and Risk. Part II: A Social Systems Perspective on the Discourses and Regulation of Hazards of Socio-Technical Systems." *Sociolagia Problemas e Practcas* 62: 97–131.

Butterworth, P., S. Schurer, T.-A. Trinh, E. Vera-Toscano, and M. Wooden. 2022. "Effect of Lockdown on Mental Health in Australia: Evidence from a Natural Experiment Analysing a Longitudinal Probability Sample Survey." *Lancet Public Health* 7 (5): E427–F436. https://doi.org/10.1016/S2468-2667(22)00082-2.

Cai, G., J. Wang, A. Lue, S. Xu, Q. Wu, K. Liu, et al. 2023. "From Pollution to Green and Low-Carbon Island Revitalization: Implications of Exhibition-Driven Sustainable Tourism for SDG 8.9 in Setouchi." *Processes* 11 (2): 623. https://doi.org/10.3390/pr11020623.

Caldarulo, M., J. Olsen, A. Frandell, S. Islam, T. P. Johnson, M. K. Feeney, et al. 2022. "COVID-19 and Gender Inequity in Science: Consistent Harm over Time." *PloS ONE* 17 (7): e0271089–e0271089. https://doi.org/10.1371/journal.pone.0271089.

Canale, N., C. Marino, M. Lenzi, A. Viento, M. D. Griffiths, M. Gabordi, et al. 2022. "How Communication Technology Fosters Individual and Social Wellbeing during the Covid-19 Pandemic: Preliminary Support for a Digital Interaction Model." *Journal of Happiness Studies* 23, 727–745. https://doi.org/10.1007/s10902-021-00421-1.

Carreras, M., S. Vera, and G. Visconti. 2023. "Who Does the Caring? Gender Disparities in COVID-19 Attitudes and Behaviours." *Politics and Gender* 19 (1): 5–33. https://doi.org/10.1017/S1743923X21000386.

Castellini, V. 2019. "Environmentalism Put to Work: Ideologies of Green Recruitment in Toronto." *Geoforum* 104: 63–70. https://doi.org/10.1016/j.geoforum.2019.06.010.

Cattivelli, V. 2023. "Macro-Regional Strategies, Climate Policies and Regional Climatic Governance in the Alps." *Climate (Basel)* 11 (2): 37. https://doi.org/10.3390/cli11020037.

Cerqua, A., and M. Letta. 2022. "Local Inequalities of the COVID-19 Crisis." *Regional Science and Urban Economics* 92: 103752–103752. https://doi.org/10.1016/j.regsciurbeco.2021.103752.

Chafi, M. B., A. Hultberg, and N. B. Yams. 2022. "Post-Pandemic Office Work: Perceived Challenges and Opportunities for a Sustainable Work Environment." *Sustainability* 14: 294. https://doi.org/10.3390/su14010294.

Chalk, J. 2021. "Neoliberalism and Personal Freedoms during COVID-19." *Journal of Global Faultlines* 8 (1): 91–99. https://doi.org/10.13169/jglobfaul.8.1.0091.

Champagne, E., A. D. Granja, and O. Choiniere. 2023. "Post-pandemic work in the public sector: A new way forward or a return to the past." *The Conversation.* https://theconversation.com/post-pandemic-work-in-the-public-sector-a-new-way-forward-or-a-return-to-the-past-204008 (accessed August 29, 2023).

Chan, S., and D. Tweedie. 2016. "Understanding Contemporary Employment Insecurity." *Work, Employment and Society* 30 (5): 896–898. https://doi.org/10.1177/0950017016644416.

Charles, L., S. Xia, and A. P. Coutts. 2022. "Digitisation and employment: A review." ILO (International Labour Organisation). https://www.ilo.org/employment/Whatwedo/Publications/WCMS_854353/lang--en/index.htm (accessed September 3, 2023).

Chatterjee, P., and A. Dev. 2023. "Labour Market Dynamics and Worker Flows in India: Impact of Covid-19." *Indian Journal of Labour Economics* 66 (1): 299–327. https://doi.org/10.1007/s41027-022-00420-7.

Chen, Z., G. Marin, D. Popp, and F. Vona. 2020. "Green Stimulus in a Post-Pandemic Recovery: The Role of Skills for a Resilient Recovery." *Environmental and Resource Economics* 76 (4): 901–911. https://doi.org/10.1007/s10640-020-00464-7.

Chen, R., M. Ramzan, M. Hafeez, and S. Ullah. 2023. "Green Innovation-Green Growth Nexus in BRICS: Does Financial Globalization Matter?" *Journal of Innovation and Knowledge* 8 (1): 100286. https://doi.org/10.1016/j.jik.2022.100286.

Chhetri, N., R. Ghimire, and D. C. Eisenhaue. 2023. "Geographies of Imaginaries and Environmental Governance." *The Professional Geographer* 75 (2): 263–268. https://doi.org/10.1080/00330124.2022.2087698.

Churchill, B. 2020. "COVID-19 and the Immediate Impact on Young People and Employment in Australia: A Gendered Analysis." *Gender, Work, and Organization.* https://doi.org/10.1111/gwao.12563.

Ciarleglio, F. A., M. Rigoni, L. Mereu, C. Tommaso, A. Carrara, G. Malossini, et al. 2021. "The Negative Effects of COVID-19 and National Lockdown on Emergency Surgery Morbidity due to Delayed Access." *World Journal of Emergency Surgery* 16 (1): 1–37. https://doi.org/10.1186/s13017-021-00382-z.

Ciravegna, L., and S. Michailova. 2022. "Why the World Economy Needs, But Will Not Get, More Globalization in the Post-COVID-19 Decade." *Journal of International Business Studies* 53: 172–186. https://doi.org/10.1057/s41267-021-00467-6.

Colin-Jaeger, N. 2021. "Reconstructing Liberalism: Hayek, Lippmann and the Making of Neoliberalism." *Oeconomia* 11 (11–2): 281–313. https://doi.org/10.4000/oeconomia.10874.

Constantinou, C. S. 2021. "People Have to Comply with the Measures: Covid-19 in 'Risk Society.'" *Journal of Applied Social Science* 15 (1): 3–11. https://doi.org/10.1177/1936724420980374.

Conti, C., M. L. Mancusi, F. Sanna-Randaccio, R. Sestini, and E. Verdolini. 2018. "Transition towards a Green Economy in Europe: Innovation and Knowledge Integration in the Renewable Energy Sector." *Research Policy* 47 (10): 1996–2009. https://doi.org/10.1016/j.respol.2018.07.007.

Contreras, F., E. Baykal, and G. Abid. 2020. "E-Leadership and Telework in Times of COVID-19 and Beyond: What We Know and Where Do We Go." *Frontiers in Psychology.* https://doi.org/10.3389/fpsyg.2020.590271.

Cooper, H., and S. Szreter. 2023. "Covid-19 and a State in Crisis: What Can the UK Learn from Its Own History?" *Cambridge Journal of Regions, Economy and Society* 16 (1): 239–244. https://doi.org/10.1093/cjres/rsac048.

Cortes, G. M., and E. Forsythe. 2023. "Heterogeneous Labor Market Impacts of the COVID-19 Pandemic." *Industrial and Labor Relations Review* 76 (1): 30–55. https://doi.org/10.1177/00197939221076856.

Cotula, L. 2021. "Towards a Political Economy of the COVID-19 Crisis: Reflections on an Agenda for Research and Action." *World Development* 138: 105235–105235. https://doi.org/10.1016/j.worlddev.2020.105235.

Crnčec, D., J. Penca, and M. Lovec. 2023. "The COVID-19 Pandemic and the EU: From a Sustainable Energy Transition to a Green Transition?" *Energy Policy* 175. https://doi.org/10.1016/j.enpol.2023.113453.

Crouch, C. 2022. "Reflections on the COVID Moment and Life Beyond Neoliberalism." *European Review of Labour and Research* 28 (1): 31–45. https://doi.org/10.1177/10242589221078125.

Croucher, G., and W. Locke. 2020. "A post-coronavirus world: Some possible trends and their implications for Australian higher education." *Melbourne CSHE.*

Discussion Paper. https://melbourne-cshe.unimelb.edu.au/__data/assets/pdf_file/0010/3371941/a-post-coronavirus-world-for-higher-education_final.pdf (accessed May 5, 2023).

Cucinotta, D., and M. Vanelli. 2020. "WHO Declares COVID-19 a Pandemic." *Acta Biomedica* 91 (1): 157–160. https://doi.org/10.23750/abm.v91i1.9397.

Dafnomilis, I., H. H. Chen, M. den Elzen, P. Fragkos, U. Chewpreecha, H. van Soest, et al. 2022. "Targeted Green Recovery Measures in a Post-COVID-19 World Enable the Energy Transition." *Frontiers in Climate* 4: 1–13. https://doi.org/10.3389/fclim.2022.840933.

Dake, K. 1992. "The Social Construction of Risk and Technology." *Journal of Social Issues* 48 (4): 21–37. https://doi.org/10.1111/j.1540-4560.1992.tb01943.x.

Damar, E. 2023. "Imagining Crises of Neoliberalism: Covid-19 Pandemic and (Im) Possibilities of Change in Turkey's Labour Regime." *Critical Sociology Eugene.* https://doi.org/10.1177/08969205231155930.

Davi, H., P.-Y. Modicom, J. L. Durand, and C. Eldin. 2021. "How Has Neoliberalism Weakened Science?" *Natures Sciences Sociétés* 3(29): 356–359. https://doi.org/10.1051/nss/2021053.

Davis, M., A. Gent, and J. Gregory. 2021. "The work-from-home technology boom." *VOXeu CEPR.* https://voxeu.org/article/work-home-technology-boon (accessed September 2, 2022).

De Groot, J., and C. Lemanski. 2021. "COVID-19 Responses: Infrastructure Inequality and Privileged Capacity to Transform Everyday Life in South Africa." *Environment and Urbanization* 33 (1): 255–272. https://doi.org/10.1177/0956247820970094.

de Miranda, K. L., and D. J. Snower. 2021. "How COVID-19 Changed the World: G-7 Evidence on a Recalibrated Relationship between Market, State, and Society." Brookings Institute. https://www.brookings.edu/research/how-covid-19-changed-the-world-g7-evidence-on-a-recalibrated-relationship-between-market-state-and-society/ (accessed September 1, 2023).

de Oliveira Neto, G. C., H. N. P. Tucci, M. G. Filho, W. C. Lucato and D. de Silva. 2022. "Moderating Effect of OHS Actions Based on WHO Recommendations to Mitigate the Effects of COVID-19 in Multinational Companies." *Process Safety and Environmental Protection: Transactions of the Institution of Chemical Engineers* 159: 652–661. https://doi.org/10.1016/j.psep.2022.01.011.

Dean, M., A. Rainnie, J. Stanford, and D. Nahum. 2021. "Industrial Policy-Making After COVID-19: Manufacturing, Innovation and Sustainability." *The Economic and Labour Relations Review: ELRR* 32 (2): 283–303. https://doi.org/10.1177/10353046211014755.

Deflem, M. 2022. "The Continuity of the Social Sciences during COVID-19: Sociology and Interdisciplinarity in Pandemic Times." *Sociology* 59: 735–746. https://doi.org/10.1007/s12115-022-00763-3.

Del Real, D., F. Crowhurst-Pons and L. Olave. 2023. "The Work, Economic, and Remittance Stress and Distress of the COVID-19 Pandemic Containment Policies: The Case of Venezuelan Migrants in Argentina and Chile." *International Journal of Environmental Research and Public Health* 20 (4): 3569. https://doi.org/10.3390/ijerph20043569.

Demena, B. A., P. A. G. van Bergeijk, and S. K. Afesorgbor. 2022. "COVID-19: The Disease of Inequality, Not Globalisation." International Institute of Social Studies. https://www.iss.nl/en/news/covid-19-disease-inequality-not-globalization (accessed September 1, 2022).

Demiralay, S., G. Gencer and F. Kilincarslan. 2023. "Risk-Return Profile of Environmentally Friendly Assets: Evidence from the NASDAQ OMX Green Economy Index Family." *Journal of Environmental Management* 337: 117683–117683. https://doi.org/10.1016/j.jenvman.2023.117683.

Dennerlein, J. T., L. Burke, E. Sabbath, J. A. R. Williams, S. E. Peters, L. Wallace, et al. 2020. "An Integrative Total Worker Health Framework for Keeping Workers Safe and Healthy during the COVID-19 Pandemic." *Human Factors: The Journal of the Human Factors and Ergonomics Society* 62 (5): 689–696. https://doi.org/10.1177/0018720820932699.

Devaraj, S., D. Faulk, M. Hicks and E. Wornell. 2021. "Globalisation, Automation and the Disruption of Local Labour Markets." In *Identifying and Managing Risk at Work: Emerging Issues in the Context of Globalisation.* Edited by C. L. Peterson, 128–142. Abingdon: Routledge.

Devlin, K., M. Fagan, and A. Connaughton, 2021. "People in Advanced Economies Say Their Society Is More Divided than Before Pandemic." Pew Research Centre. https://www.pewresearch.org/global/2021/06/23/people-in-advanced-economies-say-their-society-is-more-divided-than-before-pandemic/ (accessed August 25, 2023).

Dewey, C. 2017. "How neoliberalism has caused income inequality." *Of Course.* https://medium.com/of-course-global/how-neoliberalism-has-caused-income-inequality-9ec1fcaacb (accessed August 24, 2022).

Diffenbaugh, N. S. 2022. "COVID-19 and the Environment: Short-Run and Potential Long-Run Impacts." *Annual Review of Environment and Resources* 47 (1): 65–90. https://doi.org/10.1146/annurev-environ-120920-125207.

Digital Around the World. 2023. Data Reportal https://datareportal.com/global-digital-overview (accessed August 22, 2023).

Dinku, Y., B. Hunter, and F. Markham. 2020. "How Might COVID-19 Affect the Indigenous Labour Market." *Australian Journal of Labour Economics* 23 (2): 189–209.

Dittmer, C., and D. F. Lorenz. 2022. "A Post-COVID-19 Research Agenda for Disaster Prevention, Response and Research." In *A Research Agenda for COVID-19 and Society.* Edited by S. Matthewman, 85–103. Cheltenham: Edward Elgar Publishing.

Donelle, L., L. Comer, B. Hiebert, J. Hall, J. J. Shelley, M. J. Smith, et al. 2023. "Use of Digital Technologies for Public Health Surveillance during the COVID-19 Pandemic: A Scoping Review." *Digital Health* 9. https://doi.org/10.1177/20552076231173220.

Dorflinger, N., P. Valeria and S. Vallas. 2021. "Production Regimes and Class Compromise among European Warehouse Workers." *Work and Occupations* 48 (2): 111–145. https://doi.org/10.1177/0730888420941556.

Drotning, K. J., L. Doan, L. C. Sayer, J. N. Fish, and R. G. Rinderknecht. 2023. "Not All Homes Are Safe: Family Violence Following the Onset of the Covid-19 Pandemic." *Journal of Family Violence* 38 (2): 189–201. https://doi.org/10.1007/s10896-022-00372-y.

Du, Z., Y. Wang, Y. Bai, L. Wang, B. J. Cowling, and L. A. Meyers. 2023. "Estimate of COVID-19 Deaths, China, December 2022–February 2023." *Emerging Infectious Diseases* 29 (10): 2121–2124. https://doi.org/10.3201/eid2910.230585.

Dubey, P., G. Singh, G. Nagaraju, K. Gharat, S. D. Bharambe, and A. Vajarekar 2020. "Reduction of Workforce due to Impact of Covid-19 and Occupational Health and

Safety Management at Workplace." *International Journal of Occupational Safety and Health* 10 (2): 92–99. https://doi.org/10.3126/ijosh.v10i2.33287.

Dumont, A. M., and P. V. Baret. 2017. "Why Working Conditions Are a Key Issue of Sustainability in Agriculture? A Comparison between Agroecological, Organic and Conventional Vegetable Systems." *Journal of Rural Studies* 56: 53–64. https://doi.org/10.1016/j.jrurstud.2017.07.007.

Dütsch, M. 2022. "COVID-19 and the Labour Market: What Are the Working Conditions in Critical Jobs?" *Journal for Labour Market Research* 56 (1): 10–10. https://doi.org/10.1186/s12651-022-00315-6.

Dutta, M. J. 2020. "COVID-19, Authoritarian Neoliberalism, and Precarious Migrant Work in Singapore: Structural Violence and Communicative Inequality." *Frontiers in Communication.* https://doi.org/10.3389/fcomm.2020.00058.

Dwivedi, Y K., L. Hughes, A. K. Kar, M. Baabdullah, P. Grover, R. Abbas, et al. 2022. "Climate Change and COP26: Are Digital Technologies and Information Management Part of the Problem or the Solution? An Editorial Reflection and Call to Action." *International Journal of Information Management* 63: 102456. https://doi.org/10.1016/j.ijinfomgt.2021.102456.

Edler, S., and I. Staub. 2023. "The Impact of the Covid-19 Pandemic on Perceived Employment (In)Security in Switzerland." *Schweizerische Zeitschrift Für Soziologie* 49 (1): 179–214. https://doi.org/10.2478/sjs-2023-0010.

Edmunds, J., and B. S. Turner. 2002. *Generations, Culture and Society.* Buckingham: Open University Press. https://doi.org/10.1111/j.1468-4446.2005.00083.x.

Egana-delSol, P., G. Cruz, and A. Micco. 2022. "COVID-19 and Automation in a Developing Economy: Evidence from Chile." *Technological Forecasting and Social Change* 176: 121373–121373. https://doi.org/10.1016/j.techfore.2021.121373.

Elomäki, A., and J. Kantola. 2023. "Feminist Governance in the European Parliament: The Political Struggle over the Inclusion of Gender in the EU's COVID-19 Response." *Politics and Gender* 19 (2): 327–348. https://doi.org/10.1017/S1743923X21000544.

Engel, L., and P. Burch. 2021. "Policy Sociology in the Contemporary Global Era: Continued Importance and Pressing Methodological Considerations." *Educational Researcher* 50 (7): 474–478. https://doi.org/10.3102/0013189X211009184.

Ervasti, J., V. Aalto, J. Pentti, T. Oksanen, M. Kivimaki, and J. Vahtera. 2021. "Association of Changes in Work due to COVID-19 Pandemic with Psychosocial Work Environment and Employee Health: A Cohort Study of 24 299 Finnish Public Sector Employees." *Occupational and Environmental Medicine.* https://doi.org/10.1136/oemed-2021-107745.

Fajardo Fernández, R., R. M. Soriano-Miras, and A. Trinidad Requena. 2023. "Intersections Between the Global Economy and Gender Structures in the Workforce in Relocated Industries." *Third World Quarterly* 44 (7): 1455–1471. https://doi.org/10.1080/01436597.2023.2183835.

Farooq, F., Z. Yusop, I. S. Chaudhry, and R. Iram. 2020. "Assessing the Impacts of Globalization and Gender Parity on Economic Growth: Empirical Evidence from OIC Countries." *Environmental Science and Pollution Research International* 27 (7): 6904–6917. https://doi.org/10.1007/s11356-019-07289-y.

Farzanagan, M. R., M. Feizi, and F. Gholipor 2021. "Globalisation and the Outbreak of COVID-19: An Empirical Analysis." *Journal of Risk and Financial Management* 14: 105. https://doi.org/10.3390/jrfm14030105.

Fauser, M., A. Friedrichs, and L. Harders. 2019. "Migrations and Borders: Practices and Politics of Inclusion and Exclusion in Europe from the Nineteenth to the Twenty-First Century." *Journal of Borderlands Studies* 34 (4): 483–488. https://doi.org/10.1080/08865655.2018.1510334.

Flor, L. S., J. Friedman, C. N. Spencer, J. Cagney, A. Arrieta, M. E. Herbert, et al. 2022. "Quantifying the Effects of the COVID-19 Pandemic on Gender Equality on Health, Social, and Economic Indicators: A Comprehensive Review of Data from March 2020, to September 2021." *The Lancet (British Edition)* 399 (10344): 2381–2397. https://doi.org/10.1016/S0140-6736(22)00008-3.

Flores, N. 2013. "The Unexamined Relationship between Neoliberalism and Plurilingualism: A Cautionary Tale." *TESOL Quarterly* 47 (3): 500–520. https://doi.org/10.1002/tesq.114.

Ford, J. D., C. Zavaleta-Cortijo, T. Ainembabazi, C. Anza-Ramirez, T. Arotoma-Rojas, J. Bezerra, et al. 2022. "Interactions between Climate and COVID-19." *The Lancet: Planetary Health* 6 (10): E825–E833. https://doi.org/10.1016/S2542-5196(22)00174-7.

Forslid, R., and R. Baldwin. 2020. "COVID-19, Globotics and Development." *VOX CEPR.* https://cepr.org/voxeu/columns/covid-19-globotics-and-development (accessed August 23, 2023).

Foucault, M. (1976) 2003. "Lecture 11, 17 March 1976." In *Society Must Be Defended: Lectures at the College de France*, 239–264. New York: Picador Press.

Fradejas-García, I., J. L. Molina, and M. J. Lubbers. 2023. "Migrant Entrepreneurs in the 'Farm of Europe': The Role of Transnational Structures." *Globalizations* (ahead-of-print). 1–18. https://doi.org/10.1080/14747731.2023.2178806/

Frank, R. D. 2019. "The Social Construction of Risk in Digital Preservation." *Journal of the Association for Information Science and Technology* 71 (4): 474–484. https://doi.org/10.1002/asi.24247.

Free, C., and A. Hecimovic. 2021. "Global Supply Chains after COVID-19: The End of the Road for Neoliberal Globalisation?" *Accounting, Auditing and Accountability Journal* 34 (1). https://doi.org/10.1108/AAAJ-06-2020-4634.

Friedman, M., and R. D. Friedman. 2002. *Capitalism and Freedom*. 40th anniversary ed. Chicago: University of Chicago Press.

Frost, N. 2023. "No, 11,200 climate refugees aren't heading to Australia." *New York Times.* https://www.nytimes.com/2023/11/11/world/australia/tuvalu-climate.html#:~:text=The%20treaty%2C%20announced%20at%20the,for%20residents%20of%20the%20Pacific (accessed November 14, 2023).

Fuentes, R., M. Galeotti, A. Lanza, and B. Manzano. 2020. "COVID-19 and Climate Change: A Tale of Two Global Problems." *Sustainability* 12: 8560. https://doi.org/10.3390/su12208560.

Füleky, P., and I. Szapudi. 2022. "Bird's Eye View of COVID-19, Mobility, and Labor Market Outcomes across the US." *Economics of Disasters and Climate Change* 6 (2): 339–353. https://doi.org/10.1007/s41885-022-00110-0.

Gallistl, V., K. Bohrn, R. Rohner, and F. Kolland. 2023. "Doing Vulnerability: The Social Construction of Age(ing) during the COVID-19 Pandemic." *Zeitschrift für Gerontologie und Geriatrie* 56 (1): 18–22. https://doi.org/10.1007/s00391-022-02143-2.

Gamage, A. 2023. "Content and Process Approach to the Job Demands-Resources Model of Emotional Labour: A Conceptual Model." *Public Money and Management* 43 (5): 388–396. https://doi.org/10.1080/09540962.2021.1999596.

Gan, J., L. Liu, G Qiao, and Q. Zhang, 2023. "The Role of Robot Adoption in Green Innovation: Evidence from China." *Economic Modelling* 119: 106128. https://doi.org/10.1016/j.econmod.2022.106128.

Gandini, A. 2019. "Labour Process Theory and the Gig Economy." *Human Relations (New York)* 72 (6): 1039–1056. https://doi.org/10.1177/0018726718790002.

Gao, C., F. Zhang, D. Fang, Q. Wang, and M. Liu. 2023. "Spatial Characteristics of Change Trends of Air Pollutants in Chinese Urban Areas during 2016–2020: The Impact of Air Pollution Controls and the COVID-19 Pandemic." *Atmospheric Research* 283: 106539. https://doi.org/10.1016/j.atmosres.2022.106539.

Garel, A., and A. Petit-Romec. 2021. "Investor Rewards to Environmental Responsibility: Evidence from the COVID-19 Crisis." *Journal of Corporate Finance (Amsterdam, Netherlands)* 68: 101948–101948. https://doi.org/10.1016/j.jcorpfin.2021.101948.

Garlick, S. 2023. "Of Men and Markets: Hayek, Masculinity and Neoliberalism." *Economy and Society* 52 (1): 158–178. https://doi.org/10.1080/03085147.2022.2131273.

Gavrila, M., and M. Cilento. 2022. "Memories of the Future. Ulrich Beck, Risk and Prevention: The Difference that Defeats Indifference." *Italian Sociological Review* 12 (8S): 0_1–906. https://doi.org/10.13136/isr.v12i8S.599.

Gavriluță, N., S-P. Grecu, and H. C. Chiriac. 2022. "Sustainability and Employability in the Time of COVID-19. Youth, Education and Entrepreneurship in EU Countries." *Sustainability (Basel, Switzerland)* 14 (3): 1589. https://doi.org/10.3390/su14031589.

Geary, R. S., R. Wheeler, R. Lovell, R. Jepson, R. Hunter, and S. Rodgers. 2021. "A Call to Action: Improving Urban Green Spaces to Reduce Health Inequalities Exacerbated by COVID-19." *Preventive Medicine* 145:106425. https://doi.org/10.1016/j.ypmed.2021.106425.

Gebhard, C., V. Regitz-Zagrosek, H. K. Neuhauser, R. Morgan, and S. L. Klein. 2020. "Impact of Sex and Gender on COVID-19 Outcomes in Europe." *Biology of Sex Differences* 11: 29. https://doi.org/10.1186/s13293-020-00304-9.

Gerada, C. 2020. "Some Good Must Come Out of COVID-19." *BMJ* 369: m2043–m2043. https://doi.org/10.1136/bmj.m2043.

German Working Time Survey. 2019. https://www.infas.de/panelstudien/working-time-reporting-for-germany/?lang=en (accessed January 4, 2024).

Gheorghiev, O. 2023. "Economic Migrants in the Czech Segmented Labour Market: Covid-19 as a Magnifying Glass." *International Journal of Sociology and Social Policy* 43 (3/4): 370–383. https://doi.org/10.1108/IJSSP-06-2022-0162.

Giddens, A. 1991. *Modernity and Self Identity: Self and Society in the Late Modern Age*. Stanford: Stanford University Press.

Giddens, A. 1992. *The Transformation of Intimacy: Sexuality, Love and Emotion in Modern Societies*. Stanford: Stanford University Press.

Giddens, A. 2000. "Anthony Giddens discusses the globalisation debate." *Carnegie Endowment for International Peace*. https://carnegieendowment.org/2000/07/05/anthony-giddens-discusses-globalization-debate-pub-8655 (accessed September 1, 2023).

Gilfillan, G. 2020. "COVID-19: Labour market impact on demographic groups, industries and regions." *Parliament of Australia*. October. https://www.aph.gov.au/About_Parliament/Parliamentary_Departments/Parliamentary_Library/pubs/rp/rp2021/COVID-19-Stat_Snapshot (accessed September 10, 2022).

Gille, Z., and S. O. Riain. 2002. "Global Ethnography." *Annual Review of Sociology* 28 (1): 271–295. https://doi.org/10.1146/annurev.soc.28.110601.140945.

Giroux, H. A. 2021. "The COVID-19 Pandemic Is Exposing the Plague of Neoliberalism 1." In *Collaborative Futures in Qualitative Inquiry: Research in a Pandemic*. Edited by N. K. Denzin and M. D. Giardina, 1–11. New York: Routledge. 10.4324/9781003154587.

Godderis, L., and J. Luyten. 2020. "Challenges and Opportunities for Occupational Health and Safety after the COVID-19 Lockdowns." *Occupational and Environmental Medicine*. https://doi.org/10.1136/oemed-2020-106645.

Goffman, E. 2020. "In the Wake of COVID-19, Is Glocalization Our Sustainability Future?" *Sustainability: Science, Practice and Policy* 16 (1): 48–52. https://doi.org/10.1080/15487733.2020.1765678.

Gold, D., S. Hughes, and D. Thomas. 2021. "Perceptions, Experiences and Opportunities for Occupational Safety and Health Professionals Arising Out of the COVID-19 Pandemic." *Humanities and Social Sciences Communication* 8: 271 https://doi.org/10.1057/s41599-021-00955-y.

Goldschmidt, K. 2020. "The COVID-19 Pandemic: Technology Use to Support the Wellbeing of Children." *Journal of Paediatric Nursing* 53: 88–90. https://doi.org/10.1016/j.pedn.2020.04.013.

Goods, C. 2011. "Labour Unions, the Environment and 'Green Jobs.'" *Journal of Australian Political Economy* 67: 47–67.

Gouzoulis, G., and G. Galanis. 2021. "The Impact of Financialisaton on Public Health in Times of COVID-19 and Beyond." *Sociology of Health and Illness*. https://doi.org/10.1111/1467-9566.13305.

Grammes, N., D. Millenaar, T Fehlmann, F. Kern, M. Böhm, F. Mahfoud, et al. 2020. "Research Output and International Cooperation among Countries during the COVID-19 Pandemic: Scientometric Analysis." *Journal of Medical Internet Research* 22 (12): e24514. https://doi.org/10.2196/24514.

Gray, R. 2020. "Can the world emerge from the pandemic a better place?" *Horizon (EU Commission)*. https://ec.europa.eu/research-and-innovation/en/horizon-magazine/can-world-emerge-pandemic-better-place (accessed September 29, 2022).

Gross, T. 2023 "How 'modern Day slavery' in the Congo Powers the Rechargable Battery Economy." *Goats and Soda*. https://www.npr.org/sections/goatsandsoda/2023/02/01/1152893248/red-cobalt-congo-drc-mining-siddharth-kara (accessed September 15, 2023).

Groutsis, D., A. Kaabel, and C. F. Wright. 2023. "Temporary Migrants as Dehumanised 'Other' in the Time of COVID-19: We're All in This Together?" *Work, Employment and Society* 95001702211427. https://doi.org/10.1177/09500170221142723.

Guillen-Royo, M. 2022. "Flying Less, Mobility Practices, and Well-Being: Lessons from the COVID-19 Pandemic in Norway." *Sustainability: Science, Practice, and Policy* 18 (1): 278–291. https://doi.org/10.1080/15487733.2022.2043682.

Guivent, J. S. 2016. "Ulich Beck's Legacy." *Ambiente and Sociedade* 19 (1): 227–238. https://doi.org/10.1590/1809-4422ASOC150001ExV1912016.

Gulley, A. L. 2023. "China, the Democratic Republic of the Congo, and Artisanal Cobalt Mining from 2000 Through 2020." *Proceedings of the National Academy of Sciences – PNAS* 120 (26), e2212037120–e2212037120. https://doi.org/10.1073/pnas.2212037120

Gulmez, D. B. 2017. "Globalization." In *The Wiley Blackwell Encyclopedia of Social Theory*. Edited by B. S. Turner, 1–10. Chichester: John Wiley & Sons. https://doi.org/10.1002/9781118430873.est0842.

Ha, T. 2023. "The Disproportionate Effect of COVID-19 on the Labour Market in South Korea." *Journal of the Asia Pacific Economy*. https://doi.org/10.1080/13547860.2023.2215121.

Haberland, H. 2009. "English – The Language of Globalism." *Rask* 30: 17–45.

Hailu, D., M. Benayew, T. Liknaw, M. Ayenew, A. F. Ayalew, B. Ayano, et al. 2021. "Occupational Health Safety of Health Professionals and Associated Factors during COVID-19 Pandemics at North Showa Zone, Oromia Regional State, Ethiopia." *Risk Management and Healthcare Policy* 14: 1299–1310. https://doi.org/10.2147/RMHP.S292830.

Hall, S. 2022. "Neoliberalism and the Opportunodemic." *Journal of Extreme Anthropology* 6 (2): https://doi.org/10.5617/jea.9940.

Hall-Quinlan, D. L., H. He, X. Ren, T. P. Canty, R. J. Salawitch, P. Stratton, et al. 2023. "Inferred Vehicular Emissions at a Near-Road Site: Impacts of COVID-19 Restrictions, Traffic Patterns, and Ambient Air Temperature." *Atmospheric Environment (1994)* 299: 119649–119649. https://doi.org/10.1016/j.atmosenv.2023.119649.

Hanna, E., G. Martin, A. Campbell, P. Connolly, K. Fearon, and S. Markham. 2022. "Experiences of Face Mask Use during the COVID-19 Pandemic: A Qualitative Study." *Sociology of Health and Illness* 1–19. https://doi.org/10.1111/1467-9566.13525.

Hanna, R., Y. Xu, and D. G. Victor. 2020. "After COVID-19, Green Investment Must Deliver Jobs to Get Political Traction." *Nature (London)* 582 (7811): 178–180. https://doi.org/10.1038/d41586-020-01682-1.

Hantrais, L., J. Brannen, N. Le Feuvre, and M-T. Letablier. 2022. "Editorial: Families and COVID-19: An Interactive Relationship." *Frontiers in Sociology*. https://doi.org/10.3389/fsoc.2022.841518.

Harrell, M., S. A. Selvaraj, and M. Edgar. 2020. "DANGER! Crisis Health Workers at Risk." *International Journal of Environmental Research and Public Health* 17: 5270. https://doi.org/10.3390/ijerph17155270.

Hayek, F. A. von. 1945. "The Use of Knowledge in Society." *The American Economic Review* 35 (4): 519–530.

Hayek, F. A. von. 1948. *Individualism and Economic Order*. Chicago: University of Chicago Press.

Hean, O., and N. Chairassamee. 2023. "The Effects of the COVID-19 Pandemic on U.S. Entrepreneurship." *Letters in Spatial and Resource Sciences* 16 (1): 1–1. https://doi.org/10.1007/s12076-023-00327-x.

Heenan, N., and A. Sturman. 2020. "Labour, Nature, Capitalism and COVID-19." *The Journal of Australian Political Economy* 85: 193–199.

Hiscott, J., M. Alexandridi, M. Muscolini, E. Tassone, E. Palermo, M. Soultsioti, et al. 2020. "The Global Impact of the Coronavirus Pandemic." *Cytokine Growth Factor Review* 53: 1–9. https://doi.org/10.1016/j.cytogfr.2020.05.010.

Hodder, A. 2020. "New Technology, Work and Employment in the Era of COVID-19: Reflecting on Legacies of Research." *New Technology Work and Employment* 35 (3): 262–275. https://doi.org/10.1111/ntwe.12173.

Hoffmann, M., and R. Paulsen. 2020. "Resolving the 'Jobs-Environment-Dilemma'? The Case for Critiques of Work in Sustainability Research." *Environmental Sociology* 6 (4): 343–354. https://doi.org/10.1080/23251042.2020.1790718.

Holland, P., C. Brewster, and N. Kouglannou. 2021. "Employment, Work and Industrial Revolutions: A Faustian Deal." In *Identifying and Managing Risk at Work: Emerging Issues in the Context of Globalisation*. Edited by C. L. Peterson, 112–125. Abingdon: Routledge. https://doi.org/10.4324/9781003164029-8.

Horgen, D., J. Hackett, C. B. Westphalen, D. Kaltra, E. Richer, M. Romao, et al. 2020."Digitisation and COVID-29: The Perfect Storm." *Biomedicine Hub* 5 (3): https://doi.org/ 10.1159/000511232.

Hossain, M. F., Y. Shi, and M. Jahan. 2023. "Coronavirus (COVID-19) Pandemic Crisis Narratives and Social Construction of Risk: Comparative Case Studies of China and India." *Millennial Asia*. https://doi.org/10.1177/09763996231174268.

HSE (Health and Safety Executive). 2022. "Coronavirus (COVID-19) – Advice for workplaces." July. https://www.hse.gov.uk/coronavirus/ (accessed September 29, 2022).

Hu, Z., and S. Zhu. 2023. "Impact of the COVID-19 Outbreak on China's Tourism Economy and Green Finance Efficiency." *Environmental Science and Pollution Research International* 30 (17): 49963–49979. https://doi.org/10.1007/s11356-023-25406-w.

Hulme, M. 2010. "Cosmopolitan Climates: Hybridity, Foresight and Meaning." *Theory, Culture and Society* 27 (2–3): 267–276. https://doi.org/10.1177/0263276409358730.

Hunt, T., and H. Connolly. 2023. "Covid-19 and the Work of Trade Unions: Adaptation, Transition and Renewal." *Industrial Relations Journal* 54 (2): 150–166. https://doi.org/10.1111/irj.12395.

Hupkau, C., J. Ruiz-Valenzuela, I. E. Isphording, and S. Machin. 2023. "Labour Market Shocks and Parental Investments during the Covid-19 Pandemic." *Labour Economics* 82: 102341–102341. https://doi.org/10.1016/j.labeco.2023.102341.

Hwang, K., and S. A. Papuga. 2023. "COVID-19 Pandemic Underscores Role of Green Space in Urban Carbon Dynamics." *The Science of the Total Environment* 859 (Pt 1): 160249–160249. https://doi.org/10.1016/j.scitotenv.2022.160249.

Iavicoli, S., F. Boccuni, G. Buresti, D. Gagliardi, B. Persechino, A. Valenti, et al. 2021. "Risk Assessment at Work and Prevention Strategies on COVID-19 in Italy." *PloS ONE* https://doi.org/10.1371/journal.pone.0248874.

Ibanescu, B.-C., M. Cristea, A. Gheorghiu, and G. C. Pascariu. 2023. "The Regional Evolution of Job Insecurity during the First COVID-19 Wave in Relation to the Pandemic Intensity." *Letters in Spatial and Resource Sciences* 16 (1): 13–13. https://doi.org/10.1007/s12076-023-00337-9.

Ibled, C. 2023. "The 'Optimistic Cruelty' of Hayek's Market Order: Neoliberalism, Pain and Social Selection." *Theory, Culture and Society* 40 (3): 81–101. https://doi.org/10.1177/02632764221126305.

Igarashi, Y., S. Tateishi, T. Sawajima, K. Kikuchi, M. Kawasumi, J. Matsuoka, et al. 2022. "What Is the Role of Occupational Physicians in the Workplace during the COVID-19 Pandemic in Japan? A Qualitative Interview Study." *BMC Health Services Research* 22: 1294. https://doi.org/10.1186/s12913-022-08659-y.

ILO (International Labour Organisation). 2018. "Employment and the role of workers and employers in a green economy." In World Employment Social Outlook. *ILO*. https://onlinelibrary.wiley.com/doi/pdf/10.1002/wow3.139 (accessed July 20, 2021).

ILO (International Labour Organisation). 2020a "Psychosocial risk and work-related stress." https://www.ilo.org/safework/areasofwork/workplace-health-promotion-and-well-being/WCMS_108557/lang--en/index.htm (accessed September 26, 2022).

ILO (International Labour Organisation). 2020b. "The world of work and COVID-19." Policy Brief. *United Nations* June. https://www.ilo.org/employment/Informationresources/covid-19/other/WCMS_748323?lang=en (accessed September 20, 2022).

ILO (International Labour Organisation). 2022. "Capacity building and knowledge tour of green jobs and just transitions for government and farmer communities in Thailand." https://www.ilo.org/asia/media-centre/news/WCMS_863406/lang--en/index.htm (accessed September 18, 2023).

ILO (International Labour Organisation). 2023a. "Green jobs." https://www.ilo.org/global/topics/green-jobs/lang--en/index.htm (accessed May 23, 2023).

ILO (International Labour Organisation). 2023b. "World employment and social outlook: Trends." *ILO*. https://www.ilo.org/global/research/global-reports/weso/WCMS_865332/lang--en/index.htm (accessed May 29, 2023).

ILO (International Labour Organisation). 2023c. "Economic slowdown likely to force workers to accept lower quality jobs." *ILO*. https://www.ilo.org/global/about-the-ilo/newsroom/news/WCMS_865256/lang--en/index.htm (accessed May 29, 2023).

Imran, Z. A., and M. Ahad. 2023. "Safe-Haven Properties of Green Bonds for Industrial Sectors (GICS) in the United States: Evidence from Covid-19 Pandemic and Global Financial Crisis." *Renewable Energy* 210: 408–423. https://doi.org/10.1016/j.renene.2023.04.033.

Isakovic, N. P. 2021. "COVID-19: What has COVID-19 taught us about neoliberalism?" *Women's International League for Peace and Freedom*. https://www.wilpf.org/covid-19-what-has-covid-19-taught-us-about-neoliberalism/ (accessed September 25, 2022).

Jarvis, D. S. L. 2008. "Ulrich Beck, globalization and the rise of the risk society: A critical exegetic analysis." *Lee Kuan Yew School of Public Policy*. Research Paper No. LKYSPP08-003. https://doi.org/10.2139/ssrn.1162662 (accessed June 25, 2022).

Jarvis, D. S. L. 2021. "Work, Risk and Academic Labour: Guildism, Managerialism and the Neoliberal University." In *Identifying and Managing Risk at Work: Emerging Issues in the Context of Globalisation*. Edited by C. L. Peterson, 157–172. Abingdon: Routledge. https://doi.org/10.4324/9781003164029-11.

Jaumotte, F., L. Li, A. Medici, M. Oikonomou, C. Pizzinelli, I. Shibata, et al. 2023. "Digitisation during the COVID-19 crisis: Implications for productivity and labor markets in advanced economies." *International Monetary Fund*. https://www.imf.org/en/Publications/Staff-Discussion-Notes/Issues/2023/03/13/Digitalization-During-the-COVID-19-Crisis-Implications-for-Productivity-and-Labor-Markets-529852 (accessed May 3, 2023).

Jaworsky, B.N, and R. Qiaoan. 2021."The Politics of Blaming: the Narrative Battle between China and the US over COVID-19."*Journal of Chinese Political Science* 26: 295–315. https://doi.org/10.1007/s11366-020-09690-8.

Jeanne, L., S. Bourdin, F. Nadou, and G. Noiret. 2022 "Economic Globalization and the COVID-19 Pandemic: Global Spread and Inequalities." *GeoJournal*. https://doi.org/10.1007/s10708-022-10607-6.

Jiang, P., J. J. Klemes, Y. V. Fan, X. Fu, and Y. M. Bee. 2021."More Is Not Enough: A Deeper Understanding of the COVID-19 Impacts on Healthcare, Energy and Environment Is Needed." *International Journal of Environmental Research and Public Health* 18: 684. https://doi.org/10.3390/ijerph18020684.

Jin, J.-M., P. Bai, W. He, F. Wu, X-F. Liu, D-M. Han, et al. 2020. "Gender Differences in Patients with COVID-19: Focus on Severity and Mortality." *Frontiers in Public Health* 8: 152–152. https://doi.org/10.3389/fpubh.2020.00152.

Joby, J., and R. Thakur. 2021. "Long Term Effects of Service Adaptations Made Under Pandemic Conditions: The New 'Post COVID-19' Normal." *European Journal of Marketing* 55 (6): 1679–1700. https://doi.org/10.1108/EJM-08-2020-0607.

Jones, L., and S. Hameiri. 2021. "COVID-19 and the Failure of the Neoliberal Regulatory State." *Review of International Political Economy*. https://doi.org/10.1080/09692290.2021.1892798.

Jones, L., D. Palumbo, and D. Brown. 2021. "Coronavirus: How the pandemic has changed the world economy." *BBC News*. https://www.bbc.com/news/business-51706225 (accessed May 5, 2023).

Jong, A. 2022. "World Risk Society and Constructing Cosmopolitan Realities: A Bourdieusian Critique of Risk Society." *Frontiers of Sociology* 7. https://doi.org/10.3389/fsoc.2022.797321.

Juranek, S., J. Paetzold, H. Winner, and F. Zoutman. 2021. "Labor Market Effects of COVID-19 in Sweden and Its Neighbours: Evidence from Administrative Data." *Kyklos* 74: 512–526. https://doi.org/10.1111/kykl.12282.

Kana, M. A., R. LaPorte, and A. Jaye. 2021. "Africa's Contribution to the Science of the COVID-19/SARS-CoV-2 Pandemic." *BMJ Global Health* 6: e004059. https://doi.org/10.1136/bmjgh-2020-004059.

Kapadia, F. 2023. "Environmental Justice from Pennsylvania to Paris: A Public Health of Consequence." *American Journal of Public Health (1971)* 113 (1): 12–14. https://doi.org/10.2105/AJPH.2022.307156.

Kaplan, S., J. Lefler, and D. Zilberman. 2022. "The Political Economy of COVID-19." *Applied Economic Perspectives and Policy* 44 (1): 477–488. https://doi.org/10.1002/aepp.13164.

Karabulut, G., K. F. Zimmermann, M. H. Bilgin, and A. C. Doker. 2021. "Democracy and COVID-19 Outcomes." *Economics Letters* 203: 109840—109840. https://doi.org/10.1016/j.econlet.2021.109840.

Katz, I. T., R. Weintraub, L.-G. Bekker, and A. M. Brandt. 2021. "From Vaccine Nationalism to Vaccine Equity — Finding a Path Forward." *The New England Journal of Medicine* 384 (14): 1281–1283. https://doi.org/10.1056/NEJMp2103614.

Khama, A. 2020. "Impact of Migration of Labour Force due to Global COVID-19 Pandemic with Reference to India." *Journal of Health Management*. 22 (2): https://doi.org/10.1177/0972063420935542.

Khedhiri, S. 2023. "The Impact of COVID-19 on Agricultural Market Integration in Eastern Canada." *Regional Science Policy and Practice* 15 (2): 371–386. https://doi.org/10.1111/rsp3.12633.

Khurana, S., A. Haleem, S. Luthra, D. Huisingh, and B. Mannan. 2021. "Now Is the Time to Press the Reset Button: Helping India's Companies to Become More Resilient and Effective in Overcoming the Impacts of COVID-19, Climate Changes and Other Crises." *Journal of Cleaner Production* 280: 124466–124466. https://doi.org/10.1016/j.jclepro.2020.124466.

Kim, S.-Y., and J. E. Yang. 2023. "Psychosocial Stressors of COVID-19- and Non-COVID-19-Dedicated Nurses: A Comparative Study." *Journal of Psychosocial Nursing and Mental Health Services* 61 (1): 39–46. https://doi.org/10.3928/02793695-20220804-01.

Kirby, T. 2022. "Marion Koopmans—Preparing for the Next Pandemic." *The Lancet Infectious Diseases* 22 (5): 601–601. https://doi.org/10.1016/S1473-3099(22)00242-0.

Kitkowska, A., A. S. Alaqra, and E. Wästlund. 2023. "Lockdown Locomotion: The Fast-Forwarding Effects of Technology Use on Digital Well-Being due to COVID-19 Restrictions." *Behaviour and Information Technology* (ahead-of-print) 1–28. https://doi.org/10.1080/0144929X.2023.2203268.

Klein, J., and K. Hossain. 2020. "Conceptualising Human-Centric Cyber Security in the Arctic in the Light of Digitisation and Climate Change." *Artic Review of Law and Politics* 11: 1–18. https://doi.org/10.23865/arctic.v11.1936.

Klein, H. R., and D. L. Kleinman. 2002. "The Social Construction of Technology: Structural Considerations." *Science, Technology and Human Values* 27 (1): 28–52.

Klenert, D., F. Funke, L. Mattauch, and B. O'Callahghan. 2020. "Five Lessons from COVID-19 for Advancing Climate Change Mitigation." *Environmental and Resource Economics*. 76: 751–778. https://doi.org/10.1007/s10640-020-00453-w.

Klur, K., and S. Nies. 2023. "Governed by Digital Technology?" *Work, Organisation, Labour and Globalisation* 17 (1): 12–33. https://doi.org/10.13169/workorgalaboglob.17.1.0012.

Kodama, S. 2023. "Ethical Challenges of the COVID-19 Pandemic: A Japanese Perspective." *Journal of Medical Internet Research* 25: e44820–e44820. https://doi.org/10.2196/44820.

Koechlin, T. 2013. "The Rich Get Richer: Neoliberalism and Soaring Inequality in the United States." *Challenge* 56 (2): 5–30. https://www.jstor.org/stable/23524375.

Koh, L. Y., and K. F. Yuen. 2023. "Consumer Adoption of Autonomous Delivery Robots in Cities: Implications on Urban Planning and Design Policies." *Cities* 133: 104125. https://doi.org/10.1016/j.cities.2022.104125.

Kosoff, M. 2017. "These are the world's most serious problems, according to Millennials." *World Economic Forum Global Shapers Survey*. https://www.inc-aus.com/business-insider/worlds-top-10-problems-according-millennials-world-economic-forum-global-shapers-survey-2017.html (accessed July 31, 2023).

Kuipers, S., A. van der Witt, and J. Wolbers. 2022. "Pandemic Publishing; A Bibliometric Review of COVID-19 Research in the Crisis and Disaster Literature." *Risk Hazards and Crisis in Public Policy* 13 (4): 302–321. https://doi.org/10.1002/rhc3.12262.

Kuipers, S., and J. Wolbers. 2022. "Risk, Hazards and Crisis: Covid-19 and Beyond." *Risk, Hazards and Crisis in Public Policy* 13 (1): 6–8. https://doi.org/10.1002/rhc3.12245.

Labonté, R., G. Martin, and K. T. Storeng. 2022. "Editorial: Whither Globalization and Health in an Era of Geopolitical Uncertainty?" *Global Health* 18: 87. https://doi.org/10.1186/s12992-022-00881-x.

Lal, B., Y. K. Dwivedi, and M. Haag. 2021."Working from Home during Covid-19: Doing and Managing Technology-Enabled Social Interaction with Colleagues at a Distance." *Information Systems Frontiers*. https://doi.org/10.1007/s10796-021-10182-0.

Leahy, M. 2013. "Ulrich Beck's Cosmopolitanisation Thesis: A Philosophical Critique." *Australian Journal of Political Science* 48 (2): 152–163. https://doi.org/10.1080/10361146.2013.781115.

Lecler, R., D. Roig-Sanz, M. Puxan-Oliva, and N. Rotger. 2019. "What Makes Globalisation Really New? Sociological Views on Our Current Globalization." *Journal of Global History* 14 (3): 355–373. https://doi.org/10.1017/S1740022819000160.

Lee, S. Y. 2022. "The Political Economy of Early COVID-19 Interventions in U.S. States: Comment." *Journal of Economic Dynamics and Control* 140: 104304–104304. https://doi.org/10.1016/j.jedc.2022.104304.

Lee, T. Y., W. F. Lim, G. Y. Ang, and C. Y. Yu. 2023. "Genomic Surveillance of SARS-CoV-2 in Malaysia during the Era of Endemic COVID-19." *Life (Basel, Switzerland)* 13 (8): 1644. https://doi.org/10.3390/life13081644.

Lehberger, M., A.-K. Kleih, and K. Sparke. 2021. "Self-Reported Well-Being and the Importance of Green Spaces – A Comparison of Garden Owners and Non-Garden Owners in Times of COVID-19." *Landscape and Urban Planning* 212: 104108–104108. https://doi.org/10.1016/j.landurbplan.2021.104108.

Leppert, R. 2023. "Young workers express lower levels of job satisfaction than older ones, but most are content with their job." *Pew Research.* https://www.pewresearch.org/short-reads/2023/05/25/young-workers-express-lower-levels-of-job-satisfaction-than-older-ones-but-most-are-content-with-their-job/ (accessed October 13, 2023).

Lewis, H. 2020. "The coronavirus is a disaster for feminism." *The Atlantic.* March 2020. https://www.theatlantic.com/international/archive/2020/03/feminism-womens-rights-coronavirus-covid19/608302/ (accessed September 18, 2022).

Li, T., P. J. Barwick, Y. Deng, X. Huang, and S. Li. 2023a "The COVID-19 Pandemic and Unemployment: Evidence from Mobile Phone Data from China." *Journal of Urban Economics* 135: 103543–103543. https://doi.org/10.1016/j.jue.2023.103543

Li, L., J. Serido, R. Vosylis, A. Sorgente, Z. Lep, Y. Žhang, et al. 2023b. "Employment Disruption and Wellbeing among Young Adults: A Cross-National Study of Perceived Impact of the COVID-19 Lockdown." *Journal of Happiness Studies* 24 (3): 991–1012. https://doi.org/10.1007/s10902-023-00629-3

Liang, M., Z. Han, J. Li, Y. Sun, L. Liang, and Y Li. 2023. "Radiative Effects and Feedbacks of Anthropogenic Aerosols on Boundary Layer Meteorology and Fine Particulate Matter during the COVID-19 Lockdown over China." *The Science of the Total Environment* 862: 160767. https://doi.org/10.1016/j.scitotenv.2022.160767.

Lim, G., V. Nguyen, T. Robinson, S. Tsiaplias, and J. Wang. 2021. "The Australian Economy in 2020-21: The COVID-19 Pandemic and Prospects for Economic Recovery." *Australian Economic Review.* https://doi.org/ 10.1111/1467-8462.12405.

Liu, B., H. Chen, S. Jiang, and Q. Sun. 2021. "Why Can't I Work in a Green Way? Research on the Influencing Mechanism of Employees' Labor Intentions." *Sustainability (Basel, Switzerland)* 13 (20): 11528. https://doi.org/10.3390/su132011528.

Liu, Y., J. Zhu, C. P. Tuwor, C. Ling, L. Yu, and K. Yin. 2023. "The Impact of the COVID-19 Pandemic on Global Trade-Embodied Carbon Emissions." *Journal of Cleaner Production* 408: 137042–137042. https://doi.org/10.1016/j.jclepro.2023.137042.

Lodge, A. C., J. Earley, H. L. Peterson, P. Singh, and S. S. Manser. 2023. "Evolution of the Peer Specialist Role during COVID-19: Challenges and Opportunities for Innovation Beyond the COVID-19 Era." *Psychiatric Rehabilitation Journal.* https://doi.org/10.1037/prj0000561.

Long, E., S. Patterson, K. Maxwell, C. Blake, R. B. Perez, R. Lewis, et al. 2022. "COVID-19 Pandemic and Its Impact on Social Relationships and Health." *Journal of Epidemiology and Community Health* 76: 128–132. https://doi.org/10.1136/jech-2021-216690.

Lopez, T., T. Riedler, H. Kohnen, and M. Futterer. 2022. "Digital Value Chain Restructuring and Labour Process Transformations in the Fast-Fashion Sector: Evidence from the Value Chains of Zara & H&M." *Global Networks* 22 (4). https://doi.org/10.1111/glob.12353.

Lund, S., A. Madgavkar, J. Manyika, and S. Smit. 2020. "The Future of Remote Work: An Analysis of 2000 Tasks, 800 Jobs, and Nine Countries." McKinsey Global Institute. https://www.mckinsey.com/featured-insights/future-of-work/whats-next-for-remote-work-an-analysis-of-2000-tasks-800-jobs-and-nine-countries (accessed September 27, 2022).

Lund-Tønnesen, J., and T. Christensen. 2023. "The Dynamics of Governance Capacity and Legitimacy: The Case of a Digital Tracing Technology during the COVID-19 Pandemic." *International Public Management Journal* 26 (1): 126–144. https://doi.org/10.1080/10967494.2022.2112328.

Lupton, D. 2020. "Digital health and the coronavirus crisis: Three sociological perspectives." https://deborahalupton.medium.com/digital-health-and-the-coronavirus-crisis-three-sociological-perspectives-10ec9e01ade4 (accessed January 29, 2023).

Lupton, D. 2022a. *Covid Societies: Theorising the Coronavirus Crisis.* Abingdon: Routledge. https://doi.org/10.4324/9781003200512.

Lupton, D. 2022b. "The Quantified Pandemic: Digitised Surveillance, Containment and Care in Response to the COVID-19 Crisis." In *Everyday Automation: Experiencing an Anticipating Emerging Technologies.* Edited by S. Pink, M. Berg, D. Lupton and M. Rickenstein, 59–72. Abingdon: Routledge. https://doi.org/10.4324/9781003170884-5.

Lupu, D., and R. Tiganasu. 2022. "The Implications of Globalization on COVID-19 Vaccination in Europe." *Scientific Reports* 12 (1):17474. https://doi.org/10.1038/s41598-022-21493-w.

Lusardi, R., and S. Tomelleri. 2020. "The Juggernaut of Modernity Collapses: The Crisis of Social Planification in the Post COVID-19 Era." *Frontiers in Sociology.* https://doi.org/10.3389/fsoc.2020.611885.

MacRae, C., A. de Ruyter, J. Thompson, J. McNeill, and D. Bailey. 2021. "Brexit Risk for UK Manufacturing." In *Identifying and Managing Risk at Work: Emerging Issues in the Context of Globalisation.* Edited by C. L. Peterson, 23–36. Abingdon: Routledge. https://doi.org/10.4324/9781003164029-2.

Madgavkar, A., O. White, M. Krishnan, D. Mahajan, and X. Azcue. 2020. "COVID-19 and Gender Equality: Countering the Regressive Effects." McKinsey and Company. https://www.mckinsey.com/featured-insights/future-of-work/covid-19-and-gender-equality-countering-the-regressive-effects# (accessed September 20, 2022).

Magioglou, T., and S. Coen. 2021. "The Construction of a Hegemonic Social Representation." *European Psychologist* 26 (3): 230–240. https://doi.org/10.1027/1016-9040/a000442.

Mair, S. 2021. "Neoliberal Economics, Planetary Health, and the COVID-19 Pandemic: A Marxist Ecofeminist Analysis." *The Lancet.* https://doi.org/10.1016/S2542-5196(20)30252-7.

Maire, Q. 2023. "Towards an Historical Sociology of Global Citizenship Education Policy in Australia." *Compare* (ahead-of-print), 1–19. https://doi.org/10.1080/03057925.2023.2212108.

Maizland, L. 2023. "Global climate agreements: Successes and failures." *Council on Foreign Relations.* https://www.cfr.org/backgrounder/paris-global-climate-change-agreements (accessed November 14, 2023).

Manokha, I. 2020. "COVID-19: Teleworking, Surveillance and 24/7 Work. Some Reflections on the Expected Growth of Remote Work After the Pandemic." *Political Anthropological Research on International Social Sciences* 273–287. https://doi.org/10.1163/25903276-BJA10009.

Mansouri, F. 2020. "The sociocultural implications of COVID-19." *UNESCO.* May. https://en.unesco.org/news/socio-cultural-implications-covid-19 (accessed September 16, 2022).

Mansouri, F., and F. Sefidgarbaei. 2021. "Risk Society and COVID-19." *Canadian Journal of Public Health* 112 (1): 36–37. https://doi.org/10.17269/s41997-021-00473-z.

Manzanedo, R. D., and P. Manning. 2020. "COVID: Lessons for the Climate Change Emergency." *Science of the Total Environment* 742. https://doi.org/10.1016/j.scitotenv.2020.140563.

Margaritis, I., S. Houdart, Y. E. I. Ouadrhiri, X. Bigard, A. Vuillemin, and P. Duche. 2020. "How to Deal with COVID-19 Epidemic-Related Lockdown Physical Inactivity and Sedentary Increase in Youth? Adaptation of Anses' Benchmarks." *Archives of Public Health* 78: 52. https://doi.org/10.1186/s13690-020-00432-z.

Marital, S., and E. Barzani. 2020. "The Global Economic Impact of COVID-19: A Summary of Research." Samuel Neaman Institute for National Policy Research. https://www.neaman.org.il/Files/Global%20Economic%20Impact%20of%20COVID-19.pdf (accessed September 24, 2022).

Marston, H. R., I. Lordana, M. Fernandez-Ardevol, A. R. Climent, M. Gomez-Leon, T. D. Blanche, et al. 2020. "COVID-19: Technology, Social Connections, Loneliness, and Leisure Activities: An International Study Protocol." *Frontiers in Sociology* 5. https://doi.org/10.3389/fsoc.2020.574811.

Martell, L. 2008. "Beck's Cosmopolitan Politics." *Contemporary Politics* 14 (2): 129–143.

Martin, D., J.-L. Metzger, and P. Pierre 2006. "The Sociology of Globalization: Theoretical and Methodological Reflections." *International Sociology* 21 (4): 499–521. https://doi.org/10.1177/0268580906065298.

Marx, K. 1976. *Capital. Vol 1.* London: Penguin Books.

Marx, K. 2010. "The Process of Production of Capital." In *Collected Works.* Vol 34. *Economic Works. 1861–1864.* Edited by K. Marx and F. Engles, 339–474. London: Lawrence and Wishart.

Mathews, G. 2023. "African Trading Brokers in China: The Internet, Covid-19 and the Transformation of Low-End Globalization." *Journal of International Development* 35 (3): 491–504. https://doi.org/10.1002/jid.3654.

Ma, Z., X. Tian, and P. Zhang. 2023. "Could Ecological Restoration Reduce Income Inequality? An Analysis of 290 Chinese Prefecture-Level Cities." *Ambio* 52 (4): 802–812. https://doi.org/10.1007/s13280-022-01815-y.

Matthewman, S., and K. Huppatz. 2020. "A Sociology of COVID-19." *Journal of Sociology* 56 (4): 675–683. https://doi.org/10.1177/1440783320939416.

Mattiuzzi, C., G. Lippi, and B. M. Henry. 2021. "Healthcare Indicators Associated with COVID-19 Death Rates in the European Union." *Public Health (London)* 193: 41–42. https://doi.org/10.1016/j.puhe.2021.01.027

Maurizio, R., A. P. Monsalvo, M. S. Catania, and S. Martinez. 2023. "Short-Term Labour Transitions and Informality during the COVID-19 Pandemic in Latin America." *Journal for Labour Market Research* 57 (1): 15–15. https://doi.org/10.1186/s12651-023-00342-x.

McBride, D. 2016. "Urban Power and Community Development in the 'World Risk Society': Post-Hurricane Katrina New Orleans (usa)." *Perspectives on Global Development and Technology* 15 (1–2): 128–142. https://doi.org/10.1163/15691497-12341379.

McCausland, T. 2020. "COVID-19's Impact on Globalization and Innovation." *Research-Technology Management* 63 (6): 54–59, https://doi.org/10.1080/08956308.2020.1813506.

McClain, C., E. A. Vogels, A. Perrin, S. Sechopoulos, and L. Rainie. 2021. "The Internet and the Pandemic." The Pew Research Centre. https://www.pewresearch.org/internet/2021/09/01/the-internet-and-the-pandemic/ (accessed January 27, 2023).

McKinsey. 2021a. "To Reach the Post-COVID-19 Era, Vaccine Supply Chains Must Improve." COVID-19: Briefing note #72, September 15, 2021. McKinsey and Company. https://www.mckinsey.com/business-functions/risk-and-resilience/our-insights/covid-19-implications-for-business (accessed September 25, 2022).

McKinsey. 2021b. "COVID-19 Vaccines Demonstrate How to Achieve the Impossible." COVID-19: Briefing note #73, September 22, 2021, McKinsey and Company. https://www.mckinsey.com/business-functions/risk-and-resilience/our-insights/covid-19-implications-for-business (accessed September 25, 2022).

McKinsey 2022a. "COVID-19: Implications for Business." Briefing note #100, April 13. McKinsey and Company. https://www.mckinsey.com/capabilities/risk-and-resilience/our-insights/covid-19-implications-for-business (accessed April 22, 2023).

McKinsey. 2022b. "COVID-19: Implications for Business." Briefing note #99, April 6. McKinsey and Company. https://www.mckinsey.com/capabilities/risk-and-resilience/our-insights/covid-19-implications-for-business (accessed April 22, 2023).

McLaughlin, K. 2021. "COVID-19." Briefing note #67, August 11. McKinsey and Company. https://www.mckinsey.com/business-functions/risk-and-resilience/our-insights/covid-19-implications-for-business# (accessed September 13, 2022).

McNamara, K. R., and A. L. Newman. 2020. "The Big Reveal: COVID-19 and Globalization's Great Transformations." *International Organisation* 74: (S1): E59–E77. https://doi.org/10.1017/S0020818320000387.

Meijers, M. H., C. Scholz, R. Torfadóttir, A. Wonneberger, and M. Markov. 2022. "Learning from the COVID-19 Pandemic to Combat Climate Change: Comparing Drivers of Individual Action in Global Crises." *Journal of Environmental Studies and Sciences* 12 (4): 272–282. https://doi.org/10.1007/s13412-022-00749-x.

Mena, C., A. Karatzas, and C. Hansen. 2022. "International Trade Resilience and the Covid-19 Pandemic." *Journal of Business Research* 138: 77–91. https://doi.org/10.1016/j.jbusres.2021.08.064.

Mezzadri, A., S. Newman, and S. Stevano. 2022. "Feminist Global Political Economies of Work and Social Reproduction." *Review of International Political Economy* 29 (6): 1783–1803. https://doi.org/10.1080/09692290.2021.1957977.

Mhazo, A. T., and C. C. Maponga. 2023. "Retracing Loss of Momentum for Primary Health Care: Can Renewed Political Interest in the Context of COVID-19

Be a Turning Point?" *BMJ Global Health* 8 (7): e012668. https://doi.org/10.1136/bmjgh-2023-012668.

Michaels, D., and G. R. Wagner. 2020. "Occupational Safety and Health Administration (OSHA) and Worker Safety during the COVID-19 Pandemic." *JAMA: The Journal of the American Medical Association* 324 (14): 1389–1390. https://doi.org/10.1001/jama.2020.16343.

Milfont, T. L., D. Osborne and C. G. Sibley. 2022. "Socio-Political Efficacy Explains Increase in New Zealanders' Pro-Environmental Attitudes due to COVID-19." *Journal of Environmental Psychology* 79: 101751. https://doi.org/10.1016/j.jenvp.2021.101751.

Mishra, N. T. P., S. S. Das, S. Yadav, W. Khan, M. Afzal, A. Alarifi, et al. 2020. "Global Impacts of Pre- and Post-COVID-19 Pandemic: Focus on Socio-Economic Consequences." *Sensors International* 1. https://doi.org/10.1016/j.sintl.2020.100042.

Mo, Y., L. Deng, L. Zhang, Q., Lang, C. Liao, N. Wang, et al. 2020. "Work Stress among Chinese Nurses to Support Wuhan in Fighting against COVID-19 Epidemic." *Journal of Nursing Management* 28 (5): 1002–1009. https://doi.org/10.1111/jonm.13014.

Molino, M., E. Ingusci, F. Signori, A. Manuti, M. L. Giancaspro, V. Russo, et al. 2020. "Wellbeing Costs of Technology Use during Covid-19 Remote Working: An Investigation Using the Italian Translation of the Technostress Creators Scale." *Sustainability* 12: 5911. https://doi.org/10.3390/su12155911.

Monbiot, G. 2020. "The horror films have got it wrong: This virus has turned us into caring neighbours." *The Guardian*. 2020. https://www.theguardian.com/commentisfree/2020/mar/31/virus-neighbours-covid-19 (accessed September 25, 2022).

Montenovo, L., X. Jiang, F. Lozano-Rojas, I. Schmutte, K. Simon, K. B. A. Weinberg, et al. 2022. "Determinants of Disparities in Early COVID-19 Job Losses." *Demography* 59 (3): 827–855. https://doi.org/10.1215/00703370-9961471.

Montt, G. 2018. "Employment and the role of workers and employers in a green economy." In *World Employment Social Outlook*. ILO. https://onlinelibrary.wiley.com/doi/pdf/10.1002/wow3.139 (accessed September 26, 2022):

Moore, K., D. L. Kleinman, D. Hess, and S. Frickel. 2011. "Science and Neoliberal Globalisation: A Political Sociological Approach." *Theory and Society* 40: 505–532. https://doi.org/10.1007/s11186-011-9147-3.

Morton, J. 2020. "On the Susceptibility and Vulnerability of Agricultural Value Chains to COVID-19." *World Development* 136: 105132–105132. https://doi.org/10.1016/j.worlddev.2020.105132.

Moura de Oliveira, G., and M. Verissimo Veronese. 2023. "Brazil and the "Bolsonaro Phenomenon": Politics, the Economy, and the COVID-19 Pandemic, 2019–2020." *Latin American Perspectives*. 94582. https://doi.org/10.1177/0094582X221147597.

Mukherjee, S., and K. Pahan. 2021. "Is COVID-19 Gender-Sensitive?" *Journal of Neuroimmune Pharmacology* 16: 38–47. https://doi.org/10.1007/s11481-020-09974-z.

Mulinari, D., and K. Sandell. 2009. "A Feminist Re-reading of Theories of Late Modernity: Beck, Giddens and the Location of Gender." *Critical Sociology* 35 (4): 493–507. https://doi.org/10.1177/0896920509103980

Munawar, H. S., S. I. Khan, F. Ullah, A. Z. Kaizani, and M. A. P. Mahmud. 2021. "Effects of COVID-19 on the Australian Economy: Insights into the Mobility and Unemployment Rates in Education and Tourism Sectors." *Sustainability* 13 (20). https://doi.org/10.3390/su132011300.

Mythen, G. 2005. "From 'Goods' to 'Bads'? Revisiting the Political Economy of Risk." *Sociological Research Online* 10 (3): 1–13. https://doi.org/10.5153/sro.1140.

Mythen, G. 2021. "The Critical Theory of World Risk Society: A Retrospective Analysis." *Risk Analysis* 41 (3): 533–543. https://doi.org/10.1111/risa.13159.

Naujokaityte, G. 2020. "EU, US and China make the biggest contributions to COVID-19 research." *Science/Business*. https://sciencebusiness.net/covid-19/news-byte/eu-us-and-china-make-biggest-contributions-covid-19-research (accessed September 18, 2022).

Navarro, V. 1998. "Neoliberalism, Globalization, Unemployment, Inequalities, and the Welfare State." *International Journal of Health Services* 28 (4): 607–682. https://doi.org/10.2190/Y3X7-RG7E-6626-FVPT.

Navarro, V. 2020. "The Consequences of Neoliberalism in the Current Pandemic." *International Journal of Health Services* 50 (3): 271–275. https://doi.org/10.1177/0020731420925449.

Ndomo, Q., I. Bontenbal, and N. A. Lillie. 2023. "Essential? COVID-19 and Highly Educated Africans in Finland's Segmented Labour Market." *International Journal of Sociology and Social Policy* 43 (3/4): 339–355. https://doi.org/10.1108/IJSSP-06-2022-0171.

Neis, B., L. Butler, D. Shan, and K. Lippel. 2021. "Health and Safety Protections for the Mobile Workforce in a Pandemic: COVID-19, Globalisation and Mobilities." In *Identifying and Managing Risk at Work: Emerging Issues in the Context of Globalisation*. Edited by C. L. Peterson, 65–81. Abingdon: Routledge. https://doi.org/10.4324/9781003164029-5.

Nelkin, D. 1989. "Communicating Technological Risk: The Social Construction of Risk Perception." *Annual Review of Public Health* 10: 95–113. https://doi.org/10.1146/annurev.pu.10.050189.000523.

Newell, R., and A. Dale. 2020. "COVID-19 and Climate Change: An Integrated Perspective." *Cities and Health*. https://doi.org/10.1080/23748834.2020.1778844.

Ng, I. Y. H., Z. H. Tan, V. Chua, and A. Cheong. 2022. "Separate Lives, Uncertain Futures: Does Covid-19 Align or Differentiate the Lives of Low- and Higher-Wage Young Workers?" *Applied Research in Quality of Life* 17 (6): 3349–3380. https://doi.org/10.1007/s11482-022-10068-6.

Nga, J. L. H., W. K. Ramlan, and S. Naim. 2021. "COVID_19 Pandemic and Unemployment in Malaysia: A Case Study from Sabah." *Cosmopolitan Civil Societies: An Interdisciplinary Journal* 13 (2). http://dx.doi.org/10.5130/ccs.v13.i2.7591.

Nicolescu, V. Q., and D. E. Neaga. 2014. "Bringing the Market in, Letting the Science Out. Neoliberal Educational Reform in Romania." *Procedia – Social and Behavioural Sciences* 142: 104–110. https://doi.org/10.1016/j.sbspro.2014.07.595.

Nivakoski, S. C., X. Calo, L. Mencarini, and P. Profetta. 2022. "COVID-19 Pandemic and the Gender Divide at Work and Home." *Eurofound*. Publications Office of the European Union, Luxembourg. https://www.eurofound.europa.eu/publications/report/2022/covid-19-pandemic-and-the-gender-divide-at-work-and-home (accessed December 31, 2022).

Noh, H. S., S. Han, and Y. J. Choi. 2022. "Who Spends More to Combat COVID-19 Social Risks and Why?" *International Journal of Social Welfare* 31 (4): 392–406. https://doi.org/10.1111/ijsw.12535.

Noor, U., S. Rabbani, and G. Dastgeer. 2022. "Impact of Job Insecurity during COVID-19 on Green Entrepreneurial Intention of Pakistani Entrepreneurs: A Moderated Mediation Model." *Kybernetes*. https://doi.org/10.1108/K-11-2021-1097.

Northrup, D. 2009. "Globalization in Historical Perspective." *World Systems History. Encyclopaedia of Life Support Systems.* http://www.eolss.net/Eolss-sampleAllChapter.aspx (accessed September 27, 2022).

Nowacki, K., S. Grabowska, and K. Lakomy. 2020. "Activities of Employers and OHS Services during the Developing COVID-19 Epidemic in Poland." *Safety Science* 131. https://doi.org/10.1016/j.ssci.2020.104935.

Nygren, K. G., and A. Olofsson. 2020. "Managing the Covid-19 Pandemic Through Individual Responsibility: The Consequences of a World Risk Society and Enhanced Ethopolitics." *Journal of Risk Research* 23 (7–8):1031–1035. https://doi.org/10.1080/13669877.2020.1756382.

O'Dwyer, L. 2021. "The impact of COVID-19 on industry, innovation, skills and the need for training." *National Centre for Vocational Education Research.* Commonwealth of Australia. https://www.ncver.edu.au/__data/assets/pdf_file/0042/9667077/Impact_of_COVID_on_industry_innovation.pdf (accessed September 30, 2022).

O'Sullivan, A., J. Omukuti, and S. S. Ryder. 2023. "Global Surpluses of Extraction and Slow Climate Violence: A Sociological Framework." *Sociological Inquiry* 93 (2): 320–340. https://doi.org/10.1111/soin.12518.

O'Sullivan, D., M. Rahamathulla, and M. Pawar. 2020. "The Impact and Implications of COVID-19: An Australian Perspective." *The International Journal of Community and Social Development* 2 (2): 134–151. doi.10.1177/2516602620937922.

OECD (Organisation for Economic Cooperation and Development). 2019a. "Economic outlook: Rethink policy for a changing world." https://www.oecd.org/economic-outlook/november-2019/ (accessed June 29, 2023).

OECD (Organisation for Economic Cooperation and Development). 2019b. "Society at a glance 2019," https://www.oecd.org/social/society-at-a-glance-19991290.htm (accessed June 29, 2023).

OECD (Organisation for Economic Cooperation and Development). 2020a. "COVID-19: Protecting people and societies." https://www.oecd.org/coronavirus/policy-responses/covid-19-protecting-people-and-societies-e5c9de1a/ (accessed July 19, 2023).

OECD (Organisation for Economic Cooperation and Development). 2020b. "The territorial impact of COVID-19: Managing the crisis across levels of government." https://www.oecd.org/coronavirus/policy-responses/the-territorial-impact-of-covid-19-managing-the-crisis-across-levels-of-government-d3e314e1/ (accessed May 22, 2023).

OECD (Organisation for Economic Cooperation and Development). 2020c. "2. How COVID-19 could accelerate local labour market transitions." Job Creation and Local Economic Development. https://www.oecd-ilibrary.org/sites/a0361fec-en/index.html?itemId=/content/component/a0361fec-en (accessed September 23, 2022)

OECD (Organisation for Economic Co-operation and Development). 2021a. "The impact of COVID-19 on employment and jobs." https://www.oecd.org/employment/covid-19.htm (accessed September 23, 2022).

OECD. (Organisation for Economic Cooperation and Development). 2021b. "How will COVID_!(re-shape science, technology and innovations?" OECD

Policy Responses to coronavirus (COVID-19). https://www.oecd.org/coronavirus/policy-responses/how-will-covid-19-reshape-science-technology-and-innovation-2332334d/ (accessed January 26, 2023).

OECD (Organisation for Economic Cooperation and Development). 2021c. "The long-term environmental implications of COVID-19." OECD Policy Responses to coronavirus (COVID-19). May 2021. https://www.oecd.org/coronavirus/policy-responses/the-long-term-environmental-implications-of-covid-19-4b7a9937/ (accessed September 17, 2022).

Off, G. 2023. "Gender Equality Salience Backlash and Radical Right Voting in the Gender-Equal Context of Sweden." *West European Politics* 46 (3): 451–476. https://doi.org/10.1080/01402382.2022.2084986.

Okafor, L., and E. Yan. 2022. "Covid-19 Vaccines, Rules, Deaths, and Tourism Recovery." *Annals of Tourism Research* 95: 103424–103424. https://doi.org/10.1016/j.annals.2022.103424.

Olssen, M. 2004. "Neoliberalism, Globalisation and Democracy: Challenges for Education." *Globalisation, Societies and Education* 2 (2): 231–275. https://doi.org/10.1080/14767720410001733665.

Ongoma, V., T. E. Epule, Y. Brouziyne, M. Tanarhte, and A. Chehbouni. 2023. "COVID-19 Response in Africa: Impacts and Lessons for Environmental Management and Climate Change Adaptation." *Environment, Development and Sustainability* 1–23. https://doi.org/10.1007/s10668-023-02956-0.

Orvitz, K. 2021. "The impact of COVID-19 on workers." *OH&S (Occupational Health and Safety)*. https://ohsonline.com/articles/2021/10/01/no-title.aspx (accessed April 28, 2023).

Osler, L., and D. Zahavi. 2022. "Sociality and Embodiment: Online Communication during and after Covid-19." *Foundations of Science*. https://doi.org/10.1007/s10699-022-09861-1.

Óvári, A., A. D. Kovács, and J. Z. Farkas, 2023. "Assessment of Local Climate Strategies in Hungarian Cities." *Urban Climate* 49. https://doi.org/10.1016/j.uclim.2023.101465.

Ozili, P. 2020. "COVID-19 in Africa: Socio-Economic Impact, Policy Response and Opportunities." *International Journal of Sociology and Social Policy*. https://doi.org/10.1108/IjSSP-05-2020-0171.

Ozkan, G. 2021. "COVID-19 recovery: Some economies will take longer to rebound – this is bad for everyone." *The Conversation*. June. https://theconversation.com/covid-19-recovery-some-economies-will-take-longer-to-rebound-this-is-bad-for-everyone-162023 (accessed September 21, 2022).

Pak, A., O. A. Adegboye, A. I. Adekunie, K. M. Rahman, E. S. McBryde, and D. Eisen. 2020. "Economic Consequences of the COVID-19 Outbreak: The Need for Epidemic Preparedness." *Frontiers of Public Health*. https://doi.org/10.3389/fpubh.2020.00241.

Panday, V., A. Astha, N. Mishra, R. Greeshma, G. Lakshuana, S. Jeyavel, et al. 2021 "Do Social Connections and Digital Technologies Act as Social Cure during COVID-19?" *Frontiers in Psychology* 12. https://doi.org/10.3389/fpsyg.2021.634621.

Paremoer, L., S. Nandi, H Serag, and F. Baum. 2021." COVID-19 Pandemic and the Social Determinants of Health." *BMJ* 372: n129. https://doi.org/10.1136/bmj.n129.

Park, K.-H., A. R. Kim, M-A. Yang, S-J. Lim, and J. H. Park. 2021 "Impact of the COVID-19 Pandemic on the Lifestyle, Mental Health, and Quality of Life of Adults in South Korea." *PLoS ONE* 16 (2): e0247970. 10.1371/journal. pone.0247970.

Parker, K., J. Horowitz, and R. Minkin. 2020. "How the coronavirus outbreak has – and hasn't – changed the way Americans work." *Pew Research*. https://www. pewresearch.org/social-trends/wp-content/uploads/sites/3/2020/12/psdt_12.09.20_ covid.work_fullreport.pdf (accessed October 13, 2023).

Parwez, S. 2023. "Food for Thought: A Survey on the Nature of Work Precarity in Platform-Based On-Demand Work." *Social Policy and Society : A Journal of the Social Policy Association*. 1–17. https://doi.org/10.1017/S1474746423000015.

Patrick, F. 2013. "Neoliberalism, the Knowledge Economy and the Learner: Challenging the Inevitability of the Commodified Self as an Outcome of Education." *International Scholarly Research Notices*. https://doi.org/10.1155/2013/ 108705.

Paulsson, A., and T. Koglin. 2023. "Marketisation in Crisis: The Political Economy of COVID-19 and the Unmaking of Public Transport in Stockholm." *Critical Sociology* 49 (2): 287–303. https://doi.org/10.1177/08969205211069862.

Pauwells, L. 2019. "Exposing Globalization: Visual Approaches to Researching Connectivity in the Everyday." *International Sociology* 34 (3): 256–284. https://doi. org/10.1177/0268580919835154.

Pearman, A., M. L. Hughes, C. W. Coblenz, E. L. Smith, and S. D. Neupert. 2022. "Experiencing and Forecasting COVID-19 Daily Stress on Mental Health Reactivity across Age and Race." *The Journals of Gerontology. Series B, Psychological Sciences and Social Sciences* 77 (4): e16–e22. https://doi.org/10.1093/geronb/ gbab197.

Perkins, K. M., N. Munguia, M. Ellenbecker, R. Moure-Eraso, and L. Velazquez. 2021. "COVID-19 Pandemic Lessons to Facilitate Future Engagement in the Global Climate Crisis." *Journal of Cleaner Production* 290: 125178–125178. https://doi. org/10.1016/j.jclepro.2020.125178.

Persis, J., and A. Ben Amar. 2023. "Predictive Modeling and Analysis of Air Quality – Visualizing before and during COVID-19 Scenarios." *Journal of Environmental Management* 327: 116911–116911. https://doi.org/10.1016/j. jenvman.2022.116911.

Peters, M. A. 2021a. "The Early Origins of Neoliberalism: Colloque Walter Lippman (1938) and the Mt Perelin Society (1947)." *Educational Philosophy and Theory* https://doi.org/10.1080/00131857.2021.1951704.

Peters, M. A. 2021b. "The Disorder of Things: Quarantine Unemployment, the Decline of Neoliberalism, and the Covid-19 Lockdown Crash." *Educational Philosophy and Theory* 53 (12): 1195–1198. https://doi.org/10.1080/00131857.2020. 1759190

Peters, M. A. 2022. "Hayek as Classical Liberal Public Intellectual: Neoliberalism, the Privatization of Public Discourse and the Future of Democracy." *Educational Philosophy and Theory* 54 (5): 443–449. https://doi.org/10.1080/00131857.2019. 1696303.

Peters, S. E., J. T. Dennerlein, G. R. Warner, and G. Sorensen. 2022. "Work and Worker Health in the Post-Pandemic World: A Public Health Perspective." *The Lancet Public Health* 7 (2): E188–E194. https://doi.org/10.1016/S2468-2667(21)00259-0.

Peterson, C. L. 2018. *Stress at Work: A Sociological Perspective*. Abingdon: Routledge.

Peterson, C. L. 2021a. "Introduction: Globalisation and Risk at Work." In *Identifying and Managing Risk at Work: Emerging Issues in the Context of Globalisation*. Edited by C. L. Peterson, 3–20. Abingdon: Routledge.

Peterson, C. L., ed. 2021b. *Identifying and Managing Risk at Work: Emerging Issues in the Context of Globalisation*. Abingdon: Routledge. https://doi.org/10.4324/9781003164029.

Peterson, C. L. 2021c. "Conclusion: Globalisation, Risk and Socio-Political Contexts." In *Identifying and Managing Risk at Work: Emerging Issues in the Context of Globalisation*. Edited by C. L. Peterson, 205–218. Abingdon: Routledge. https://doi.org/10.4324/9781003164029-14.

Peterson, C. L., and C. Walker. 2022. "Universal Health Care and Political Economy, Neoliberalism and Effects of COVID-19: A View of Systems and Complexity." *Journal of Evaluation in Clinical Practice*. 28 (2): 338–340. https://doi.org/10.1111/jep.13631.

Petrović, D., M. Petrović, N. Bojković, and V. P. Čokić, 2020 "An Integrated View on Society Readiness and Initial Reaction to COVID–19: A Study across European Countries." *PLoS ONE* 15 (11): e0242838. https://doi.org/10.1371/journal.pone.0242838.

Pieterse, J. N. 2008. "Globalization the Next Round: Sociological Perspectives." *Futures* 40 (8): 707–720. https://doi.org/10.1016/j.futures.2008.02.005.

Pietrocola, M., E. Rodrigues, F. Bercot, and S. Schnorr. 2021. "Risk Society and Science Education: Lessons from the Covid-19 Pandemic." *Science Education (Dordr)* 30 (2): 209–233. https://doi.org/10.1007/s11191-020-00176-w.

Pileggi, S. F. 2021. "Life Before COVID-19: How Was the World Actually Performing?" *Quality Quantity* 55 (5):1871–1888. https://doi.org/10.1007/s11135-020-01091-6.

Piroşcă, G. I, G. L. Şerban-Oprescu, L. Badea, M.-R. Staned-Puică and C.R. Valdebenito. 2021. "Digitalization and Labor Market—A Perspective within the Framework of Pandemic Crisis" *Journal of Theoretical and Applied Electronic Commerce Research* 16 (7): 2843–2857. https://doi.org/10.3390/jtaer16070156.

Pollitt, H., R. Lewney, B. Kiss-Dobrony, and X. Lin. 2021. "Modelling the Economic Effects of COVID-19 and Possible Green Recovery Plans: A Post-Keynesian Approach." *Climate Policy* 21 (10): 1257–1271. https://doi.org/10.1080/14693062.2021.1965525.

Popescu, C. R. G., ed. 2022. *COVID-19 Pandemic Impact on New Economy Development and Societal Change*. Hershey: IGI Global. https://doi.org/10.4018/978-1-6684-3374-4.

Posocco, L., and I. Watson. 2023. "Re-Imagining the Nation-State: An Impetus from the Pandemic." *Frontiers in Sociology* 8: 1086569–1086569. https://doi.org/10.3389/fsoc.2023.1086569.

Pröbstl-Haider, U., K. Gugerell, and S. Maruthaveeran, 2023. "Covid-19 and Outdoor Recreation – Lessons Learned? Introduction to the Special Issue on 'Outdoor Recreation and Covid-19: Its Effects on People, Parks and Landscapes'." *Journal of Outdoor Recreation and Tourism* 41: 100583. https://doi.org/10.1016/j.jort.2022.100583.

Pultz, S., M. P. Hansen, and H. Jepsen. 2021. "Planning for a Job: The Trying Experience of Unemployment during the COVID-19 Crisis in Denmark." *International*

Perspectives in Psychology: Research, Practice, Consultation 10 (4): 228–242. https://doi.org/10.1027/2157-3891/a000028.

Puri, N., E. A. Coomes, H. Haghbayan, and K. Gunaratne. 2020. "Social Media and Vaccine Hesitancy: New Updates for the Era of COVID-19 and Globalized Infectious Diseases." *Human Vaccines and Immunotherapeutics* 16 (11): 2586–2593. https://doi.org/10.1080/21645515.2020.1780846.

Queen, D. 2021. "Technological Impact of COVID-19." *International Wound Journal.* 18 (2): 129–130. https://doi.org/10.1111/iwj.13578.

Quiggin, J. 1999. "Globalisation, Neoliberalism and Inequality in Australia." *The Economic and Labour Relations Review* 10 (2): 240–259. https://doi.org/10.1177/103530469901000206.

Raab, M., M. Rutland, B. Schonberger, H. P. Blossfeld, D Hofacker, S. Buchholz, et al. 2008. "GlobalIndex: A Sociological Approach to Globalization Measurement." *International Sociology* 23 (4): 596–613. https://doi.org/10.1177/0268580908090729.

Raimondi, F., L. Novelli, A. Ghirardi, F. M. Russo, D. Pellegrini, R. Biza, et al. 2021. "Covid-19 and Gender: Lower Rate But Same Mortality of Severe Disease in Women – An Observational Study." *BMC Pulmonary Medicine* 21 (1): 96–96. https://doi.org/10.1186/s12890-021-01455-0.

Ramos, D., T. Cotrim, P. Arezes, J. Baptista, M. Rodrigues, and J. Leitão. 2022. "Frontiers in Occupational Health and Safety Management." *International Journal of Environmental Research and Public Health* 19: 10759. https://doi.org/10.3390/ijerph191710759.

Rana, P., and F. Fleischman. 2023. "Indian Forest Governance during the COVID-19 Pandemic." *The International Forestry Review* 25 (1): 105–120. https://doi.org/10.1505/146554823836838727.

Ranka, S., J. Quigley, and T. Hussain. 2020. "Behaviour of Occupational Health Services during the COVID-19 Pandemic." *Occupational Medicine* 70: 359–363. https://doi.org/10.1093/occmed/kqaa085.

Rasmussen, P., J. D'warte, S. Gannon, H. R. Hansen, R. Jacobs, F. S. Knage, et al. 2023. "'Reworldings': Exploring Perspectives on the Future from Danish and Australian Youth during COVID-19." *Journal of Youth Studies*, 1–18.

Räthzel, N., and D. Uzzell. 2011. "Trade Unions and Climate Change: The Jobs Versus Environment Dilemma." *Global Environmental Change* 21 (4): 1215–1223. https://doi.org/10.1016/j.gloenvcha.2011.07.010.

Raunkiaer, M., D. S. Joergensen, A. Rasmussen, G. Johannesen, J. Thuesen, C. M. Elnegaard, et al. 2023. "Experiences of Improvement of Everyday Life Following a Rehabilitation Programme for People with Long-Term Cognitive Effects of COVID-19: Qualitative Study." *Journal of Clinical Nursing.* https://doi.org/10.1111/jocn.16739.

Reinsberg, B., A. Kentikelenis, and T. Stubbs. 2021. "Creating Crony Capitalism: Neoliberal Globalisation and the Fueling of Corruption," *Socio-Economic Review* 19 (2): 607–634. https://doi.org/10.1093/ser/mwz039.

Rezio, L., E. de Oliveira, A. M. Queiroz, de. Sousa, R. Zerbetto, P. M. Marcheti, et al. 2022. "Neoliberalism and Precarious Work in Nursing in the COVID-19 Pandemic: Repercussions on Mental Health." *Revista Da Escola de Enfermagem Da U S P* 56: e20210257–e20210257. https://doi.org/10.1590/1980-220X-REEUSP-2021-0257.

Richter, H. 2022. "COVID-19, Viral Social Theory and Immunitarian Perceptions – A Case for Postfoundational Critique." *Distinktion: Journal of Social Theory* 23 (2–3): 183–199. https://doi.org/10.1080/1600910X.2022.2099232.

Rivera-Cuadrado, W. 2023. "Healthcare Practitioners' Construction of Occupational Risk during the COVID-19 Pandemic." *Social Science & Medicine (1982)* 331: 116096–116096. https://doi.org/10.1016/j.socscimed.2023.116096.

Robertson, R., G. Lopez-Acevedo, and Y. Savchenko. 2020. "Globalisation and the Gender Earnings Gap: Evidence from Sri Lanka and Cambodia." *The Journal of Development Studies* 56 (2): 295–313. https://doi.org/10.1080/00220388.2019.1573986.

Robina-Ramírez, M., S.-O. Sánchez, H. V. Jiménez-Naranjo, and J. Castro-Serrano. 2022. "Tourism Governance during the COVID-19 Pandemic Crisis: A Proposal for a Sustainable Model to Restore the Tourism Industry." *Environment, Development and Sustainability* 24 (5): 6391–6412. https://doi.org/10.1007/s10668-021-01707-3.

Robinson, W. I. 2018. "The Next Economic Crisis: Digital Capitalism and Global Police State." *Race and Class* 60 (1): 77–92. https://doi.org/10.1177/0306396818769016.

Rodrigues, J. 2013. "The Political and Moral Economies of Neoliberalism: Mises and Hayek." *Cambridge Journal of Economics* 37 (5): 1001–1017. https://doi.org/10.1093/cje/bes091.

Rodriguez-Jimenez, R., N. E. Fares-Otero, and L. García-Fernández. 2023. "Gender-Based Violence during COVID-19 Outbreak in Spain." *Psychological Medicine* 53 (1): 299–300. https://doi.org/10.1017/S0033291720005024.

Ruiu, M. L., M. Ragnedda, and G. Ruiu. 2020. "Similarities and Differences in Managing the Covid-19 Crisis and Climate Change Risk." *Journal of Knowledge Management* 24 (10): 2597–2614. https://doi.org/10.1108/JKM-06-2020-0492.

Ryner, J. M. 2023. "Silent Revolution/Passive Revolution: Europe's COVID-19 Recovery Plan and Green Deal." *Globalizations* 20 (4): 628–643. https://doi.org/10.1080/14747731.2022.2147764.

Saad-Filho, A. 2020. "From COVID-19 to the End of Neoliberalism." *Critical Sociology* 46 (4–5): 477–485. https://doi.org/10.1177/0896920520929966.

Saad-Filho, A. 2021. "Neoliberalism and the Pandemic." *Notebooks: The Journal for Studies on Power* 1 (1): 179–186. https://doi.org/10.1163/26667185-01010010.

Saher, R., and M. Anjum. 2021. "Role of Technology in COVID-19 Pandemic." In *Researches and Applications of Artificial Intelligence to Mitigate Pandemics.* Edited by K. Hameed, S. Bhaties and S. T. Ahmed, 109–138. London: Academic Press. https://doi.org/10.1016/B978-0-323-90959-4.00005-5.

Saleem, F., M. I. Malik, and S. S. Qureshi. 2021. "Work Stress Hampering Employee Performance during COVID-19: Is Safety Culture Needed?" *Frontiers in Psychology*. https://doi.org/10.3389/fpsyg.2021.655839.

Sandbrook, C., E. Gómez-Baggethun, and W. M. Adams. 2022. "Biodiversity Conservation in a Post-COVID-19 Economy." *Oryx. 56* (2): 277–283. https://doi.org/10.1017/S0030605320001039.

Sandhu, D., and R. Barn. 2022. "'The Internet Is Keeping Me from Dying from Boredom': Understanding the Management and Social Construction of the Self Through Middle-Class Indian Children's Engagement with Digital Technologies during the COVID-19 Lockdown." *International Journal on Child Maltreatment: Research, Policy and Practice,* 1–16. https://doi.org/10.1007/s42448-022-00135-8.

Santurtún, A., and J. Shaman. 2023. "Work Accidents, Climate Change and COVID-19." *The Science of the Total Environment* 871: 162129–162129. https://doi.org/10.1016/j.scitotenv.2023.162129.

Schaupp, S. 2022. "COVID-19, Economic Crises and Digitalisation: How Algorithmic Management Became an Alternative to Automation." *New Technology, Work and Employment.* https://doi.org/10.1111/ntwe.12246.

Schöley, J., J. M. Aburto, I. Kashnitsky, M. S. Kniffka, L. Zhang, H. Jaadla, et al. 2022. "Life Expectancy Changes Since COVID-19." *Nature Human Behaviour* 6: 1649–1659. https://doi.org/10.1038/s41562-022-01450-3.

Scognamiglio, F., A. Sancino, F. Caló, C. Jacklin-Jarvis, and J. Rees. 2023. "The Public Sector and Co-Creation in Turbulent Times: A Systematic Literature Review on Robust Governance in the COVID-19 Emergency." *Public Administration (London)* 101 (1): 53–70. https://doi.org/10.1111/padm.12875.

Seetharaman, P. 2020. "Business Models Shifts: Impact of Covid-19." *International Journal of Information Management* 54: 102173–102173. https://doi.org/10.1016/j.ijinfomgt.2020.102173.

Sepadi, M. M., and V. Nkosi. 2022. "Environment and Occupational Health Exposure and Outcomes of Informal Street Food Vendors in South Africa: A Quasi-Systematic Review." *International Journal of Environmental Research and Public Health* 19 (3): 1348. https://doi.org/10.3390/ijerph19031348.

Sharior, F., M.-U. Alam, M. Zaqout, S. Cawood, S. Ferdous, D. M. Shoaib, et al. 2023 "Occupational Health and Safety Status of Waste and Sanitation Workers: A Qualitative Exploration during the COVID-19 Pandemic across Bangladesh." *PLOS Water* 2 (1): e0000041. 10.1371/journal.pwat.0000041.

Shimoni, S. 2023. "The Unprotectables: A Critical Discourse Analysis of Older People's Portrayal in UK Newspaper Coverage of Covid-19." *European Journal of Cultural Studies* https://doi.org/10.1177/13675494231185539.

Shin, H., and S. Park. 2023. "Are Firms with Women Executives Better at Surviving a Crisis? Evidence from South Korea during the COVID-19 Pandemic." *Gender in Management* 38 (1): 133–151. https://doi.org/10.1108/GM-09-2021-0279.

Shrestha, N., M. Y. Shad, O. Ulvi, M. H. Khan, A. Karamehic-Muratovic, U. D. T. Nguyen, et al. 2020 "The Impact of COVID-19 on Globalization." *One Health.* 11: 100180. https://doi.org/10.1016/j.onehlt.2020.100180.

Sideri, K., and B. Prainsack. 2023. "COVID-19 Contact Tracing Apps and the Governance of Collective Action: Social Nudges, Deliberation, and Solidarity in Europe and Beyond." *Policy Studies* 44 (1): 132–153. https://doi.org/10.1080/01442872.2022.2130884.

Silva, J. M., S. Carley, and D. M. Konisky. 2023. "'I Earned the Right to Build the Next American Car': How Autoworkers and Communities Confront Electric Vehicles." *Energy Research and Social Science* 99. https://doi.org/10.1016/j.erss.2023.103065.

Silver, L., and A. Connaughton. 2022. "Partisanship Colors Views of COVID-19 Handling across Advanced Economies." Pew Research Centre. https://www.pewresearch.org/global/2022/08/11/partisanship-colors-views-of-covid-19-handling-across-advanced-economies/ (accessed September 11, 2022).

Simon, S. 2023. "The 'Covid-Trigger': New Light on Urban Agriculture and Systemic Approach to Urbanism to Co-Create a Sustainable Lisbon." *Systemic Practice and Action Research* 36 (1): 87–109. https://doi.org/10.1007/s11213-022-09598-9.

Sims, M., P. Calder, M. Moloney, A. Rothe, M. Rogers, L. Doan, et al. 2022. "Neo-liberalism and Government Response to COVID-19: Ramifications for Early Child-hood Education and Care." *Issues in Educational Research* 32 (3): 1174–1195.

Singh, K., D. Kondal, S. Mohan, S. Jaganathan, M. Deepa, N. S. Venkateshmurthy, et al. 2021."Health, Psychosocial, and Economic Impacts of the COVID-19 Pandemic on People with Chronic Conditions in India: A Mixed Methods Study." *BMC Public Health* 21: 685. https://doi.org/10.1186/s12889-021-10708-w.

Singh, V., H. Shirazi, and J. Turetken. 2022. "COVID-19 and Gender Disparities: Labour Market Outcomes." *Research in Economics* 76 (3): 206–217. https://doi.org/10.1016/j.rie.2022.07.011.

Skelton, C. 2005. "The 'Individualized' (Woman) in the Academy: Ulrich Beck, Gender and Power." *Gender and Education* 17 (3): 319–332. https://doi.org/10.1080/09540250500145049.

Soga, M., M. J. Evans, D. T. C. Cox, and K. J. Gaston. 2021. "Impacts of the COVID-19 Pandemic on Human-Nature Interactions: Pathways, Evidence and Implications." *Perspective* 3: 518–527. https://doi.org/10.1002/pan3.10201.

Sormunen, M., L. Lattke, K. Leksy, K. Dadaczynski, E. Sakellari, V. Velasco, et al. 2022. "Health Promoting Schools and COVID-19: Preparing for the Future." *Scandinavian Journal of Public Health* 50 (6): 655–659. https://doi.org/10.1177/14034948221091155.

Sorrell, J. M. 2021. "Losing a Generation: The Impact of COVID-19 on Older Americans." *Journal of Psychosocial Nursing and Mental Health Services* 59 (4): 9–12. https://doi.org/10.3928/02793695-20210315-03.

Sowers, E. A. 2017. "Logistics Labor: Insights from the Sociologies of Globalization, the Economy, and Work." *Sociology Compass* 11 (3): e12459–n/a. https://doi.org/10.1111/soc4.12459.

Sowles, N. 2019. "Changes in Official Poverty and Inequity Rates in the Anglophone World in the Age of Neoliberalism." *Angles* 8. https://doi.org/10.4000/angles.560.

Sparke, M., and O. D. Williams. 2022. "Neoliberal Disease: COVID-19, Co-Pathogenesis and Global Health Insecurities." *Environment and Planning A: Economy and Space* 54 (1): 15–32. https://doi.org/10.1177/0308518X211048905.

Spitzer, D. L., S. Thambiah, Y. L. Wong, and M. K. Kaundan. 2023. "Globalization and the Health and Well-Being of Migrant Domestic Workers in Malaysia." *Globalization and Health*. 19 (1): 29–29. https://doi.org/10.1186/s12992-023-00925-w.

Statista. 2023. "Projected gross volume of the gig economy from 2018-2023." https://www.statista.com/statistics/1034564/gig-economy-projected-gross-volume/ (accessed September 15, 2023).

Strachan, S., A. Greig, and A. Jones. 2023. "Going Green Post COVID-19: Employer Perspectives on Skills Needs." *Local Economy*. 26909422311516. https://doi.org/10.1177/02690942231151638.

Su, C.-W., K. Dai, S. Ullah, and Z. Andlib. 2021. "COVID-19 Pandemic and Unemployment Dynamics in European Economies." *Economic Research*. https://doi.org/10.1080/1331677X.2021.1912627.

Sumonja, M. 2021. "Neoliberalism Is Not Dead: On Political Implications of COVID-19." *Capital and Class*. 45 (2). https://doi.org/10.1177/0309816820982381.

Suomi, A., T. P. Schofield, and P. S. Butterworth. 2020. "Unemployment, Employ-ability and COVID19: How the Global Socioeconomic Shock Challenged Negative Perceptions toward the Less Fortunate in the Australian Context." *Frontiers in Psychology*. https://doi.org/10.3389/fpsyg.2020.594837.

Tabbush, C. 2021. "COVID-19's social and economic fallout hits women harder." *INTER PRESS SERVICE.* June 2021. http://www.ipsnews.net/2021/01/covid-19s-social-economic-fallout-hits-women-harder/ (accessed September 26, 2022).

Thangavel, P., P. Pathak, and B. Chandra. 2021. "COVID-19: Globalisation – Will the Course Change?" *Vision: The Journal of Business Perspective.* https://doi.org/10.1177/0972262920984571.

The Conversation. 2020. "The world before this coronavirus and after cannot be the same." *The Conversation.* https://theconversation.com/the-world-before-this-coronavirus-and-after-cannot-be-the-same-134905 (accessed April 19, 2023).

The Conversation. 2023. "Global economy 2023. COVID-19 turned global supply chains upside down – 3 ways the pandemic forced companies to rethink and transform how they source their products." *The Conversation.* https://theconversation.com/global-economy-2023-covid-19-turned-global-supply-chains-upside-down-3-ways-the-pandemic-forced-companies-to-rethink-and-transform-how-they-source-their-products-196764 (accessed April 27, 2023).

The Lancet. 2023. Editorial. "The COVID-19 Pandemic in 2023: Far from Over." *The Lancet.* 401 (10371): 79. https://doi.org/10.1016/S0140-6736(23)00050-8.

Thorpe, D. 2020. "How Investing in the Green Economy Is the Best Way to Post-Covid-19 Economic Recovery." *Proceedings of the Institution of Civil Engineers. Civil Engineering* 173 (3): 100–100. https://doi.org/10.1680/jcien.2020.173.3.100.

Thorpe, C., and D. Inglis. 2019. "Do 'Global Generations' Exist?" *Youth and Globalization* 1 (1): 40–64. https://doi.org/10.1163/25895745-00101003.

Thorpe, A. K., E. A. Kort, D. H. Cusworth, A. Ayasse, B. Bue, and V. Yadav. 2023. "Methane Emissions Decline from Reduced Oil, Natural Gas, and Refinery Production during COVID-19." *Environmental Research Communications* 5 (2): 021006. https://doi.org/10.1088/2515-7620/acb5e5.

Tooze, A. 2021. "Has Covid ended the neoliberal era?" *The Guardian.* https://www.theguardian.com/news/2021/sep/02/covid-and-the-crisis-of-neoliberalism (accessed September 25, 2022).

Toquero, C. M. D., R. A. Calargo, and S. B. Pormento. 2021. "Neoliberalism Crisis and the Pitfalls and Glories in Emergency Remote Education." *Asian Journal of Distance Education* 16 (1): 90–97. https://doi.org/10.5281/zenodo.4672777.

Toshkov, D. 2023. "Explaining the Gender Gap in COVID-19 Vaccination Attitudes." *European Journal of Public Health.* https://doi.org/10.1093/eurpub/ckad052.

Toulan, O. 2020. "Globalisation after COVID-19: What's in store?" *Research and Knowledge.* May. https://www.imd.org/research-knowledge/articles/Globalization-after-COVID-19-Whats-in-store/ (accessed September 20, 2022).

Turner, B. S. 2010a. "Reflexive Traditionalism and Emergent Cosmopolitanism: Some Reflections on the Religious Imagination." *Soziale Welt* 61 (3/4): 313–318. https://doi.org/10.5771/0038-6073-2010-3-4-313.

Turner, B. S. 2010b. "Theories of Globalization: Issues and Origins." In *The Routledge International Handbook of Globalization Studies.* Edited by B. S. Turner, 3–22. Abingdon: Routledge. https://doi.org/10.4324/9781315867847.

Tušl, M., R. Brauchli, P. Kerksieck, and G. F. Bauer. 2021. "Impact of the COVID-19 Crisis on Work and Private Life, Mental Well-Being and Self-Rated Health in German and Swiss Employees: A Cross-Sectional Online Survey." *BMC Public Health* 21: 741. https://doi.org/10.1186/s12889-021-10788-8.

Tweedie, D., and S. Chan. 2021. "Precarious Work and Globalisation in Australia: Growth, Risks and Future(s)." In *Identifying and Managing Risk at Work:*

Emerging Issues in the Context of Globalisation. Edited by C. L. Peterson, 82–95. Abingdon: Routledge. https://doi.org/10.4324/9781003164029-6.

Tyler, I. 2015. "Classificatory Struggles: Class, Culture and Inequality in Neoliberal Times." *The Sociological Review* 63 (2): 493–511. https://doi.org/10.1111/1467-954X.12296.

Ulceluse, M., and F. Bender, F. 2022. "Two-Tier EU Citizenship: Disposable Eastern European Workers during the COVID-19 Pandemic." *Organization (London, England)* 29 (3): 449–459. https://doi.org/10.1177/13505084211061229.

Ullah, A. K. M. A., S. N. H. Alkaff, S. C. W. Lee, D. Chattoraj, and J. Ferdous. 2023. "Globalization and Migration: The Great Gender Equalizer?" *Journal of International Women's Studies* 25 (3): 1–16. https://doi.org/10.1080/13545701.2012.688998.

UN (United Nations). 2021. "What combatting COVID-19 can teach us about tackling the climate crisis." *United Nations Academic Impact.* https://www.un.org/en/academic-impact/what-combating-covid-19-can-teach-us-about-tackling-climate-crisis (accessed September 25, 2022).

UN (United Nations). 2023a. "The Paris agreement: What is the Paris agreement?" *UN Climate Change.* https://unfccc.int/process-and-meetings/the-paris-agreement (accessed May, 12 2023).

UN (United Nations). 2023b. "Climate Action." https://www.un.org/sustainabledevelopment/climate-action/ (accessed May 16, 2023).

Vargo, D., L. Zho, B. Benwell, and Z. Yan. 2020. "Digital Technology Use during COVID-19 Pandemic: A Rapid Review." *Human Behaviour and Emerging Technologies* 3 (1): 13–24. https://doi.org/10.1002/hbe2.242.

Vecchione, M., and F. Lucidi. 2022. "Basic Personal Values in the Midst of the COVID-19 Pandemic in Italy: A Two-Wave Longitudinal Study." *PloS ONE* 17 (9): e0274111–e0274111. https://doi.org/10.1371/journal.pone.0274111.

Venugopal, R. 2015. "Neoliberalism as Concept". *Economy and Society* 44 (2): 165–187. https://doi.org/10.1080/03085147.2015.1013356.

Verschuur, J., E. E. Koks, and J. W. Hall. 2021. "Global Economic Impacts of COVID-19 Lockdown Measures Stand Out in High-Frequency Shipping Data." *PLoS ONE* 16 (4): e0248818. https://doi.org/10.1371/journal.pone.0248818.

Vilanova, R., E. Miranda, and I. Martins. 2021. "Neoliberalism and Science Education South of the Equator: Perspectives from Brazil." *Cultural Studies of Science Education* 16: 1069–1081. https://doi.org/10.1007/s11422-021-10041-z.

Vogel, K. D., M. F. Johnson, and A. G. Sveinsdóttir. 2023. "Communities at Risk for Mobilization: Neoliberal Governance and the (Un)Contentious Politics of the Dakota Access Pipeline in Rural Illinois." *Journal of Rural Studies* 99: 134–143. https://doi.org/10.1016/j.jrurstud.2023.02.013.

Vyas, L. 2022. "'New Normal' at Work in a Post-COVID World: Work–Life Balance and Labor Markets." *Policy and Society* 41 (1):155–167. https://doi.org/10.1093/polsoc/puab011.

Vyas, L., and N. Butakhieo 2021. "The Impact of Working from Home during COVID-19 on Work and Life Domains: An Exploratory Study on Hong Kong." *Policy Design and Practice* 4 (1): 59–76. https://doi.org/10.1080/25741292.2020.1863560.

Wahaj, Z., M. M. Alam and A. Q. Al-Amin. 2022." Climate Change and COVID-19: Shared Challenges, Divergent Perspectives, and Proposed Collaborative Solutions." *Environmental Science and Pollution Research International* 29 (11): 16739–16748. https://doi.org/10.1007/s11356-021-18402-5.

Walby, S. 2021. "The COVID Pandemic and Social Theory: Social Democracy and Public Health in the Crisis." *European Journal of Social Theory* 24 (1): 22–43. https://doi.org/10.1177/1368431020970127.

Walker, C. 2021. "Climate Change and Risk to Workers: Piecing Together the Puzzle." In *Identifying and Managing Risk at Work: Emerging Issues in the Context of Globalisation*. Edited by C. L. Peterson, 99–111. Abingdon: Routledge. https://doi.org/10.4324/9781003164029-7.

Walker, C., and C. L. Peterson. 2021. "Universal Health Coverage and Primary Health Care: Their Place in People's Health." *Journal of Evaluation in Clinical Practice* 27 (5): 1027–1032. https://doi.org/10.1111/jep.13445.

Wang, D., and Z. Mao. 2021. "From Risks to Catastrophes: How Chinese Newspapers Framed the Coronavirus Disease 2019 (COVID-19) in Its Early Stage." *Health, Risk and Society* 23 (3–4): 93–110. https://doi.org/10.1080/13698575.2021.1901859.

Ward, P. R. 2020. "A Sociology of the COVID-19 Pandemic: A Commentary and Research Agenda for Sociologists." *Journal of Sociology* 56 (4): 726–735. https://doi.org/10.1177/1440783320939682.

Washif, J. A., A. Ammar, K. Trabelsi, K. Chamari, C. S. M. Chong, S. F. A. Mohd Kassim, et al. 2021. "Regression Analysis of Perceived Stress among Elite Athletes from Changes in Diet, Routine and Well-Being: Effects of the COVID-19 Lockdown and 'Bubble' Training Camps." *International Journal of Environmental Research and Public Health* 19 (1): 402. https://doi.org/10.3390/ijerph19010402.

Watson, I. 2016. "Wage Inequality and Neoliberalism: The Australian Experience." *Journal of Industrial Relations*. 58 (1): 131–149. https://doi.org/10.1177/0022185615598191.

Watson, R., Z. W. Kundzewicz, and L. Borrell-Damián. 2022. "Covid-19, and the Climate Change and Biodiversity Emergencies." *The Science of the Total Environment* 844: 157188–157188. https://doi.org/10.1016/j.scitotenv.2022.157188.

Watterson, A. 2020." COVID-19 in the UK and Occupational Health and Safety: Predictable Not Inevitable Failures by Government, and Trade Union and Nongovernmental Organization Responses." *NEW SOLUTIONS: A Journal of Environmental and Occupational Health Policy* 30 (2): 86–94. https://doi.org/10.1177/1048291120929763.

Weber, M. 2001 *The Protestant Ethic and the Spirit of Capitalism*. London: Routledge. https://doi.org/10.4324/9780203995808.

WEF (World Economic Forum). 2019. "The global risks report." 14th ed. https://www3.weforum.org/docs/WEF_Global_Risks_Report_2019.pdf (accessed July 31, 2023).

Weinberger, B. 2021. "Vaccination of Older Adults: Influenza, Pneumococcal Disease, Herpes Zoster, COVID-19 and Beyond." *Immunity and Ageing* 18 (1): 1–38. https://doi.org/10.1186/s12979-021-00249-6.

Weins, N. W., A. L. Zhu, J. Qian, F. Barbi Seleguim, and I. da Costa Ferreira. 2023. "Ecological Civilization in the Making: the 'Construction' of China's Climate-Forestry Nexus." *Environmental Sociology* 9 (1): 6–19. https://doi.org/10.1080/23251042.2022.2124623.

WHO (World Health Organisation). 2020a. "WHO Director-General's opening remarks at the media briefing on COVID-19 – 11 March 2020." https://www.who.int/director-general/speeches/detail/who-director-general-s-opening-remarks-at-the-media-briefing-on-covid-19---11-march-2020 (accessed October 16, 2023).

WHO (World Health Organisation). 2020b."Impact of COVID-19 on people's livelihoods, their health and our food system." https://www.who.int/news/item/13-10-2020-impact-of-covid-19-on-people's-livelihoods-their-health-and-our-food-systems#:~:text=The%20economic%20and%20social%20disruption,the%20end%20of%20the%20year. (accessed April 22, 2023).

WHO (World Health Organisation). 2021a. "COVID-19: Occupational health and safety for health workers: interim guidance, 2 February." https://www.who.int/publications/i/item/WHO-2019-nCoV-HCW_advice-2021-1 (accessed September 21, 2022).

WHO (World Health Organisation). 2021b. "A global study of digital crisis interaction among GenZ and Millennials." https://www.who.int/news-room/feature-stories/detail/social-media-covid-19-a-global-study-of-digital-crisis-interaction-among-gen-z-and-millennials (accessed January 31, 2023).

WHO (World Health Organisation). 2023a. "WHO Coronavirus (COVID-19) Dashboard." https://covid19.who.int/ (accessed December 24, 2023).

WHO (World Health Organisation). 2023b. "The true death toll of COVID-19." https://www.who.int/data/stories/the-true-death-toll-of-covid-19-estimating-global-excess-mortality (accessed April 14, 2023).

WHO (World Health Organisation). 2023c. "Coronavirus disease (COVID-19)." https://www.who.int/health-topics/coronavirus#tab=tab_1 (accessed April 24, 2023).

Williamson, J. G. 1996. "Globalisation, Convergence and History." *Journal of Economic History* 56 (2): 277–306. https://doi.org/10.1017/S0022050700016454.

Winder, G. 2011. "Market Solutions." In *Revisiting Risk Society: A Conversation with Ulrich Beck*. Rachael Carsons Center for Environment and Society. Edited by L. Culver, H. Egner, S. Gallini, A. Kneitz, C. Lousley, U. Lubken, et al. 15–17. Munich. https://www.environmentandsociety.org/sites/default/files/2011_6_risk_society.pdf (accessed April 25, 2023).

Woods, T., D. Schneider, and K. Harknett. 2023. "The Politics of Prevention: Polarization in How Workplace COVID-19 Safety Practices Shaped the Well-Being of Frontline Service Sector Workers." *Work and Occupations* 50 (1): 130–162. https://doi.org/10.1177/07308884221125821.

Working Time Survey for Germany. 2019. https://www.infas.de/panelstudien/working-time-reporting-for-germany/?lang=en (accessed January 1, 2024).

Wu, F., G. Tang, and W. Sun. 2018. "Exploring 'New Generation' Employees' Green Tactics in Environmental Protection in China." *Asia Pacific Business Review* 24 (4): 510–527. https://doi.org/10.1080/13602381.2018.1451131.

Wu, Y., and H. Mustafa. 2023. "Exploring the Impact of Social Media Exposure Patterns on People's Belief in Fake News during COVID-19: A Cross-Gender Study." *Online Journal of Communication and Media Technologies* 13 (3): e202326. https://doi.org/10.30935/ojcmt/13117.

Xames, M. D., J. Shefa, and F. Sarwar. 2023. "Bicycle Industry as a Post-Pandemic Green Recovery Driver in an Emerging Economy: A SWOT Analysis." *Environmental Science and Pollution Research International* 30 (22): 61511–61522. https://doi.org/ 10.1007/s11356-022-21985-2.

Xu, L., Z. Yang, J. Chen, and Z. Zou. 2023. "Impacts of the COVID-19 Epidemic on Carbon Emissions from International Shipping." *Marine Pollution Bulletin* 189: 114730–114730. https://doi.org/10.1016/j.marpolbul.2023.114730.

Xuan, X., K. Khan, C. W. Su, and A. Khurshid. 2021. "Will COVID-19 Threaten the Survival of the Airline Industry?" *Sustainability (Basel, Switzerland)* 13 (21): 11666. https://doi.org/10.3390/su132111666.

Yang, Z. 2023. "How did China come to dominate the world of electric cars?" *MIT Technology Review.* https://www.technologyreview.com/2023/02/21/1068880/how-did-china-dominate-electric-cars-policy/ (accessed September 18, 2023).

Yang, H., C. Krantzberg, X. Dong, and X. Hu. 2023. "Environmental Outcomes of Climate Migration and Local Governance: An Empirical Study of Ontario." *International Journal of Climate Change Strategies and Management* 15 (3): 371–390. https://doi.org/10.1108/IJCCSM-07-2022-0081.

Yao, Z., Y. Wang, X. Qiu, and F. Song. 2023. "Impact of Anthropogenic Emission Reduction during COVID-19 on Air Quality in Nanjing, China." *Atmosphere* 14 (4): 630. https://doi.org/10.3390/atmos14040630.

Yaya, S., A. Otu, and R. Labonté. 2020. "Globalisation in the Time of COVID-19: Repositioning Africa to Meet the Immediate and Remote Challenges." *Global Health* 16: 51. https://doi.org/10.1186/s12992-020-00581-4.

Yoshimitsu, T. 2020. "COVID-19 and a better model for society: How globalization and urbanization created the perfect storm." *Nippon.Com.* https://www.nippon.com/en/in-depth/d00610/ (accessed September 26, 2022).

Yu, X., Y. Li, C. Hu, H. Xu, X. Zhao, and J. Huang. 2020. "Factors Associated with Job Satisfaction of Frontline Medical Staff Fighting against COVID-19: A Cross-Sectional Study in China" *Frontiers in Public Health. Occupational Health and Safety.* https://doi.org/10.3389/fpubh.2020.00426.

Yu, X., H. Song, T. Ren, and Y. Xue. 2023. "COVID-19 and Labour Market Resilience: Evidence from Large-Scale Recruitment Behaviour." *Regional Studies* 58 (1): 45–60. https://doi.org/10.1080/00343404.2023.2181325.

Yuan, Z., Y. Xiao, Z. Dai, J. Huang, Z. Zhang, and Y. Chen. 2020. "Modelling the Effects of Wuhan's Lockdown during COVID-19, China." *Bulletin of the World Health Organization* 98 (7): 484–494. https://doi.org/10.2471/BLT.20.254045.

Zaman, A., and J. Das. 2020. "Injustice Versus Insecurity: Climate-Induced Displacement in the Fijian and New Zealand Public Discourses." *Pacific Journalism Review: PJR* 26 (2): 102–117. https://doi.org/10.24135/pjr.v26i2.1098.

Zang, S., X. Zhang, Y. Xing, J. Chen, L. Lin, and Z. Hou. 2023. "Applications of Social Media and Digital Technologies in COVID-19 Vaccination: Scoping Review." *Journal of Medical Internet Research* 25: e40057–e40057. https://doi.org/10.2196/40057.

Zarocostas, J. 2023. "Increasing Humanitarian Concerns for 2023." *The Lancet (British Edition)* 401 (10370): 13–14. https://doi.org/10.1016/S0140-6736(22)02587-9.

Zemmar, A., A. M. Lozano, and B. J. Nelson. 2020. "The Rise of Robots in Surgical Environments during COVID-19." *Perspectives* 2: 566–572. https://doi.org/10.1038/s42256-020-00238-2.

Zeuner, B. 2018. "An Obsolescing Bargain in a Rentier State: Multinationals, Artisanal Miners, and Cobalt in the Democratic Republic of Congo." *Frontiers in Energy Research* 6. https://doi.org/10.3389/fenrg.2018.00123.

Zhang, J., M. Ahmad, T. Muhammad, F. Syed, X. Hong, and M. Khan. 2023b. "The Impact of the Financial Industry and Globalization on Environmental Quality." *Sustainability (Basel, Switzerland)* 15 (2): 1705. https://doi.org/10.3390/su15021705.

Zhang, T., R. Banerjee, and A. Amarshi. 2023. "Does Canada's Express Entry System Meet the Challenges of the Labor Market?" *Journal of Immigrant and Refugee Studies* 21 (1): 104–118. https://doi.org/10.1080/15562948.2022.2133201.

Zhang, Y., F. Sun, Z. Huang, L. Song, S. Jin and L. Chen. 2023a. "Predicting the Impact of the COVID-19 Pandemic on Globalisation." *Journal of Cleaner Production* 409: 137173–137173. https://doi.org/10.1016/j.jclepro.2023.137173.

Zheng, X., Y. Lu, C. Ma, J. Yuan, N. C. Stenseth, D. O. Hessen, et al. 2023. "Greenhouse Gas Emissions from Extractive Industries in a Globalized Era." *Journal of Environmental Management* 343: 118172–118172. https://doi.org/10.1016/j.jenvman.2023.118172.

Zhou, Y. R. 2022 "Vaccine Nationalism: Contested Relationships between COVID-19 and Globalization," *Globalizations* 19 (3): 450–465. https://doi.org/10.1080/14747731.2021.1963202.

Zimmermann, B. M., K. T. Paul, E. R. Araújo, A. Buyx, S. Ferstl, A. Fiske, et al. 2023a. "The Social and Socio-Political Embeddedness of COVID-19 Vaccination Decision-Making: A Five-Country Qualitative Interview Study from Europe." *Vaccine* 41 (12): 2084–2092. https://doi.org/10.1016/j.vaccine.2023.02.012.

Zimmermann, T., S. Shinde, D. Parthasarathy, and N. Narayanan. 2023b. "Linking Climate Change Adaptation and Disaster Risk Reduction: Reconceptualizing Flood Risk Governance in Mumbai." *Journal of Integrative Environmental Sciences* 20 (1): 1–29. https://doi.org/10.1080/1943815X.2023.2169712.

Zulver, J. M., T. P. Cookson, and L. Fuentes. 2021. "COVID-19 and Gender-Based Violence: Reflections from a 'Data for Development' Project on the Colombia-Venezuela Border." *International Feminist Journal of Politics* 23 (2): 341–349. https://doi.org/10.1080/14616742.2021.1894208.

Zungu, M., K. Voyi, M. N. langeni, S. V. Moodley, J. Ramodike, N. Claassen, et al. 2021. "Organizational Factors Associated with Health Worker Protection during the COVID-19 Pandemic in Four Provinces of South Africa." *BMC Health Services Research* 21: 1080. https://doi.org/10.1186/s12913-021-07077-w.

Zyoud, S. H. 2021. "The Arab Region's Contribution to Global COVID-19 Research: Bibliometric and Visualization Analysis." *Global Health* 17 (31). https://doi.org/10.1186/s12992-021-00690-8.

Index

For Product Safety Concerns and Information please contact our EU
representative GPSR@taylorandfrancis.com
Taylor & Francis Verlag GmbH, Kaufingerstraße 24, 80331 München, Germany

9 781032 582849